The 100 Most Influential MEDICAL PIONEERS OF ALL TIME

THE BRITANNICA GUIDE TO THE
WORLD'S MOST INFLUENTIAL PEOPLE

THE 100 MOST INFLUENTIAL
MEDICAL
PIONEERS
OF ALL TIME

EDITED BY MONICA K. GILL

Britannica
Educational Publishing

IN ASSOCIATION WITH

ROSEN
EDUCATIONAL SERVICES

Published in 2017 by Britannica Educational Publishing (a trademark of Encyclopædia Britannica, Inc.) in association with The Rosen Publishing Group, Inc.
29 East 21st Street, New York, NY 10010

Copyright © 2017 by Encyclopædia Britannica, Inc. Britannica, Encyclopædia Britannica, and the Thistle logo are registered trademarks of Encyclopædia Britannica, Inc. All rights reserved.

Rosen Publishing materials copyright © 2017 The Rosen Publishing Group, Inc. All rights reserved.

Distributed exclusively by Rosen Publishing.
To see additional Britannica Educational Publishing titles, go to rosenpublishing.com.

First Edition

Britannica Educational Publishing
J.E. Luebering: Executive Director, Core Editorial
Anthony L. Green: Editor, Compton's by Britannica

Rosen Publishing
Monica K. Gill: Editor
Nelson Sá: Art Director
Michael Moy: Designer
Cindy Reiman: Photography Manager
Carina Finn: Photo Researcher

Library of Congress Cataloging-in-Publication Data

Names: Gill, Monica K., editor.
Title: The 100 most influential medical pioneers of all time / edited by Monica K. Gill.
Other titles: One hundred most influential medical pioneers of all time
Description: First edition. | New York : Britannica Educational Publishing, 2017. | Series: The Britannica guide to the world's most influential people | Includes bibliographical references and index.
Identifiers: LCCN 2015034140 | ISBN 9781680482812 (library bound : alk. paper)
Subjects: LCSH: Medicine—History—Encyclopedias.
Classification: LCC R125 .A13 2016 | DDC 610.3—dc23
LC record available at http://lccn.loc.gov/2015034140

Manufactured in China

Photo credits:
Cover, p. 3 Nonwarit/Shutterstock.com; pp. 8, 304, 308, 310 wongwean/Shutterstock.com; pp. 10-11, 46, 254, 269 Science Source; p. 24 DEA Picture Library/De Agostini/Getty Images; p. 33 Sheila Terry/Science Source; pp. 64, 72, 113, 177 Courtesy of the National Library of Medicine; p. 84, 147 Photos.com/Thinkstock; p. 102 Universal Images Group/Getty Images; p. 126 Cassell & Company/Library of Congress, Washington, D.C. (LC-DIG-pga-00466); p. 139 Library of Congress Prints and Photographs Division; p. 187 © Alamy; p. 191 ullstein bild/Getty Images; p. 224 Library of Congress, Washington, D.C. (neg. no. LC USZ 62 058326); p. 226 Library of Congress, Washington, D.C. (LC-DIG-ppmsca-07205); p. 233 Bain News Service/Library of Congress, Washington, D.C. (LC-DIG-ggbain-23218); p. 239 science photo/Shutterstock.com; p. 250 Francis Miller/The LIFE Picture Collection/Getty Images; p. 258 Mondadori/Getty Images; p. 260 Al Ravenna-World Journal Tribune/Library of Congress, Washington, D.C. (dig. id. cph 3c31540); p. 284 Andreas Feininger/The LIFE Picture Collection/Getty Images; p. 289 Thos Robinson/Getty Images Entertainment/Getty Images; p. 294 Pascal Le Segretain/Getty Images; p. 295 Alex Wong/Getty Images; p. 301 The Asahi Shimbun/Getty Image

CONTENTS

Introduction	8
Imhotep	23
Hippocrates	25
Pedanius Dioscorides	31
Galen of Pergamum	32
Hua Tuo	38
al-Rāzī	40
Avicenna	41
Moses Maimonides	51
Paracelsus	56
Ambroise Paré	61
Andreas Vesalius	62
Gabriel Fallopius	66
William Harvey	67
Thomas Sydenham	76
Marcello Malpighi	78
Antonie van Leeuwenhoek	82
William Cheselden	87
Sir Percivall Pott	88
James Lind	91
John Hunter	93
William Withering	94
Benjamin Rush	97
Edward Jenner	99
René-Théophile-Hyacinthe Laënnec	104
François Magendie	108
John Snow	109
Ann Preston	112
Horace Wells	114
Ignaz Philipp Semmelweis	115
Mayo Family	119
William Thomas Green Morton	122

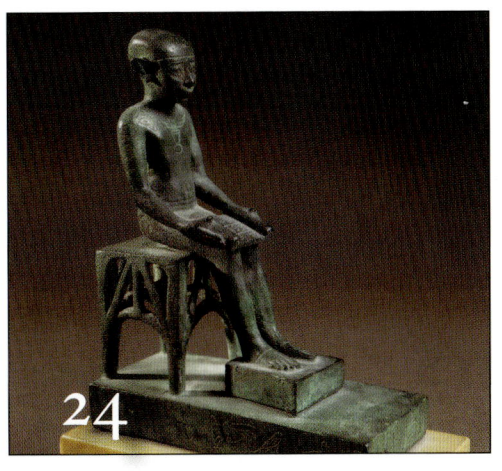

24

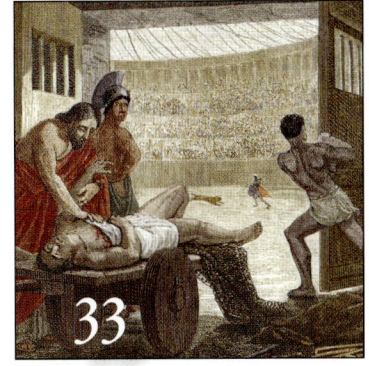

33

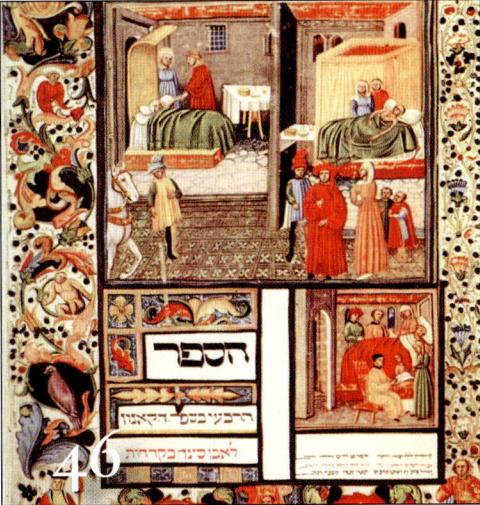

46

Florence Nightingale	123
Elizabeth Blackwell	129
Rudolf Virchow	131
Clara Barton	138
Louis Pasteur	141
Joseph Lister, Baron Lister of Lyme Regis	153
Emeline Horton Cleveland	158
Rebecca Lee Crumpler	159
Mary Jane Safford	160
Mary Putnam Jacobi	162
Robert Koch	164
Wilhelm Conrad Röntgen	170
Alphonse Laveran	171
William Osler	173
Walter Reed	176
Santiago Ramón y Cajal	180
Kitasato Shibasaburo	181
Paul Ehrlich	183
Emil von Behring	189
Sigmund Freud	190
Daniel Hale Williams	214
Rebecca Lee Dorsey	215
William Bateson	216
Abraham Flexner	218
Karl Landsteiner	219
Florence Rena Sabin	221
Sara Josephine Baker	223
Carl Jung	225
Oswald Avery	230
Margaret Sanger	232
Marie Stopes	235
Alexander Fleming	236
Selman Abraham Waksman	241
Frederick Grant Banting	242
Helen Brooke Taussig	244
Howard Walter Florey	246
Charles Best	247

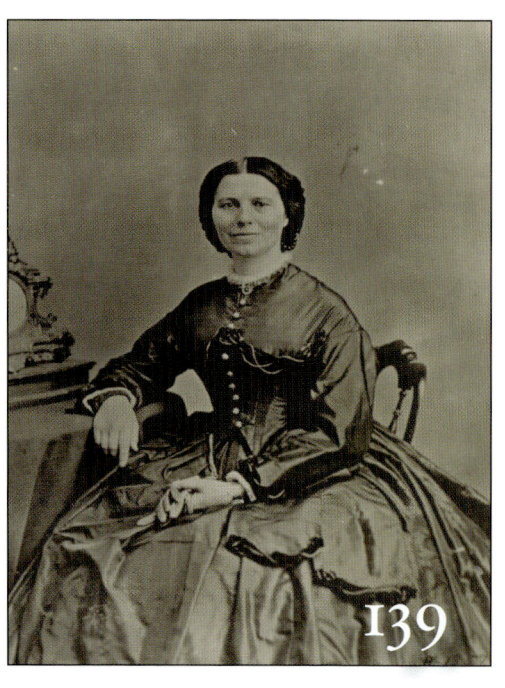

139

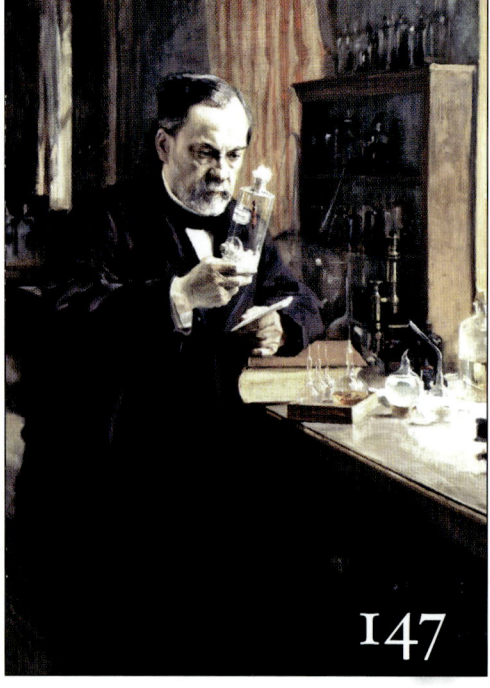

147

Alfred Blalock	248
Percy Julian	249
Barbara McClintock	251
Charles Richard Drew	253
Ernst Boris Chain	255
Albert Sabin	256
Rita Levi-Montalcini	257
Virginia Apgar	259
Paul Maurice Zoll	262
Jonas Salk	263
Francis Harry Compton Crick	265
Adrian Kantrowitz	267
Joseph E. Murray	268
Rosalind Franklin	269
Denton A. Cooley	271
Rosalyn S. Yalow	271
Christiaan Barnard	273
Stanley Cohen	275
Alexander Gordon Bearn	276
Roger Charles Louis Guillemin	279
Baruch S. Blumberg	280
Andrew V. Schally	281
James Dewey Watson	282
Luc Montagnier	285
Oliver Sacks	286
J. Michael Bishop	290
Harald zur Hausen	292
Harold Varmus	292
Francoise Barré-Sinoussi	294
Francis Collins	295
James Thomson	298
Shinya Yamanaka	300
Glossary	304
For Further Reading	308
Index	310

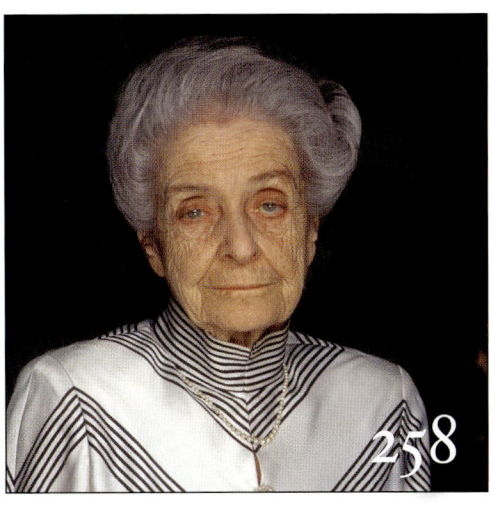

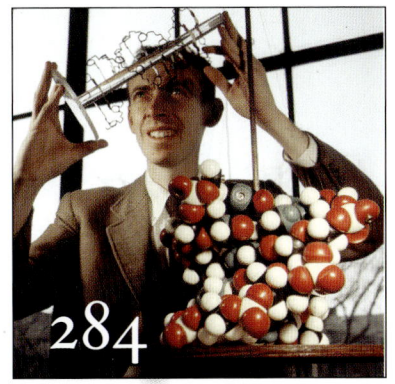

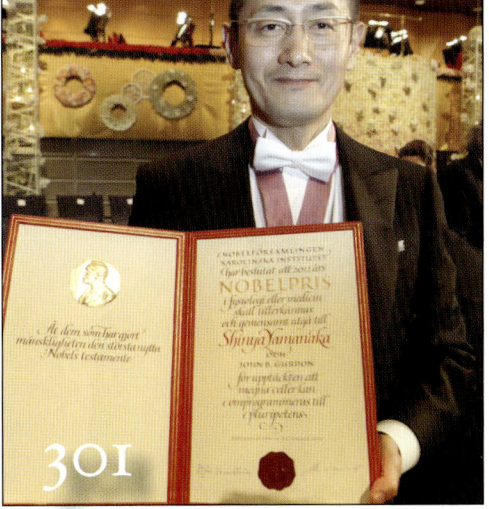

Introduction

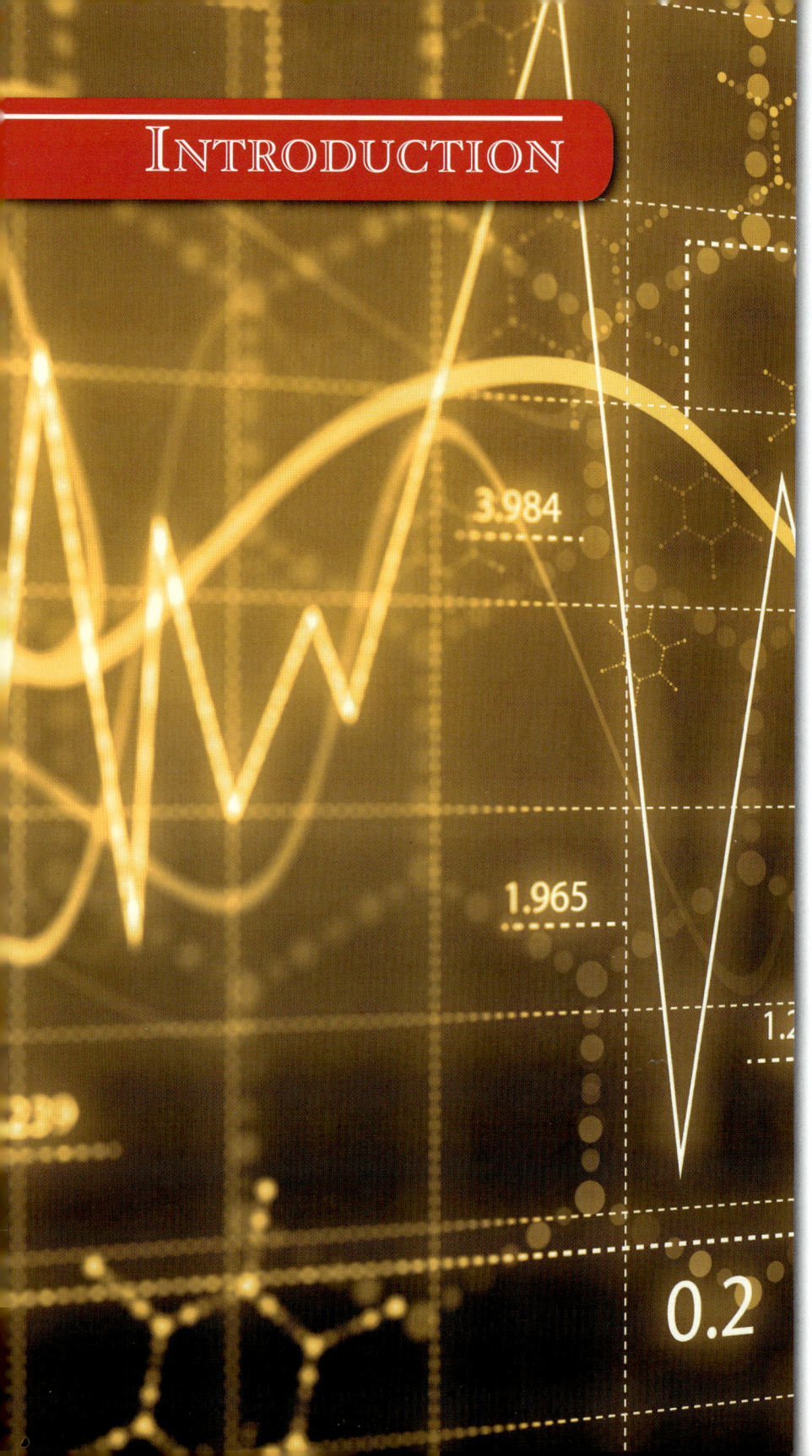

Introduction

The practice of medicine—the science and art of preventing, alleviating, and curing disease—is one of the oldest professional callings. Since ancient times, healers with varying degrees of knowledge and skills have sought to restore the health or relieve the distress of the sick and injured. Often, that meant doing little more than offering sympathy to the patient while nature took its course. Today, however, practitioners of medicine have several millennia of medical advances on which to base their care of patients.

Evidence of attempts to care for the sick and injured predates written records. Skulls found in Europe and South America dating as far back as 10,000 BCE have shown that the practice of trepanning, or trephining (removal of a portion of the skull bone), was not uncommon. This operation, performed by many early peoples, including American Indians, was probably done to release evil spirits that were thought to be the source of illness; yet, in many cases, it proved to be the medically correct thing to do. Opening the skull can relieve pressure and pain caused by brain tumours and head injuries.

Indeed, much of early medicine was closely identified with pagan religions and superstitions. Illness was attributed to angry gods or evil spirits; prayers, incantations, and other rituals were used to appease the gods or ward off demons—and thereby drive off disease. Nonetheless, the ancients did not entirely lack valid medical knowledge. In fact, through observation and experience, they acquired considerable wisdom about sickness and its prevention and relief.

The book of Leviticus in the Old Testament described quarantine regulations and sanitary practices that were used to prevent the spread of leprosy and plague. The ancient Romans realized the importance of sanitation to

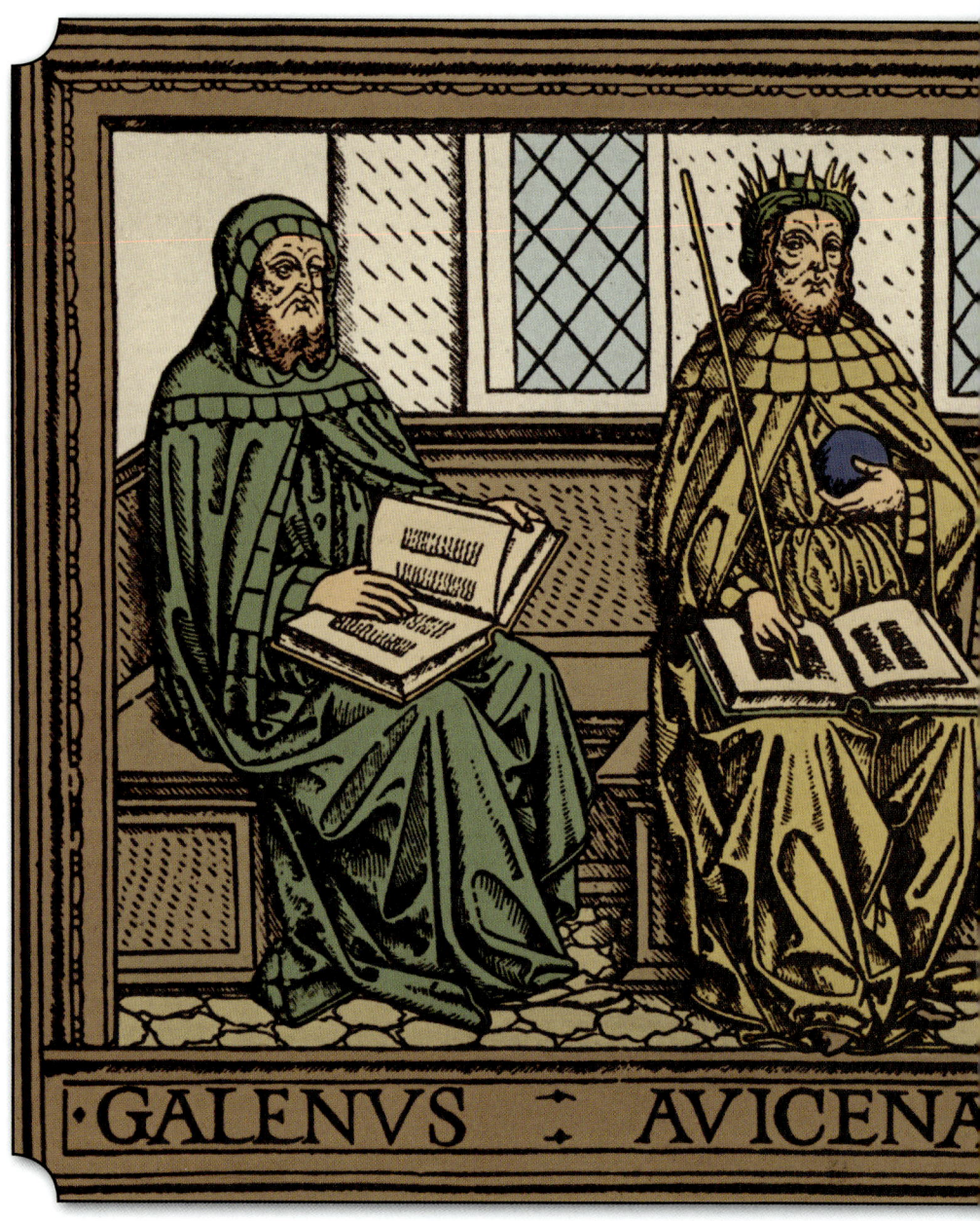

Galen (left), *Avicenna* (centre), *and Hippocrates are three of the great figures of ancient medicine.*

Introduction

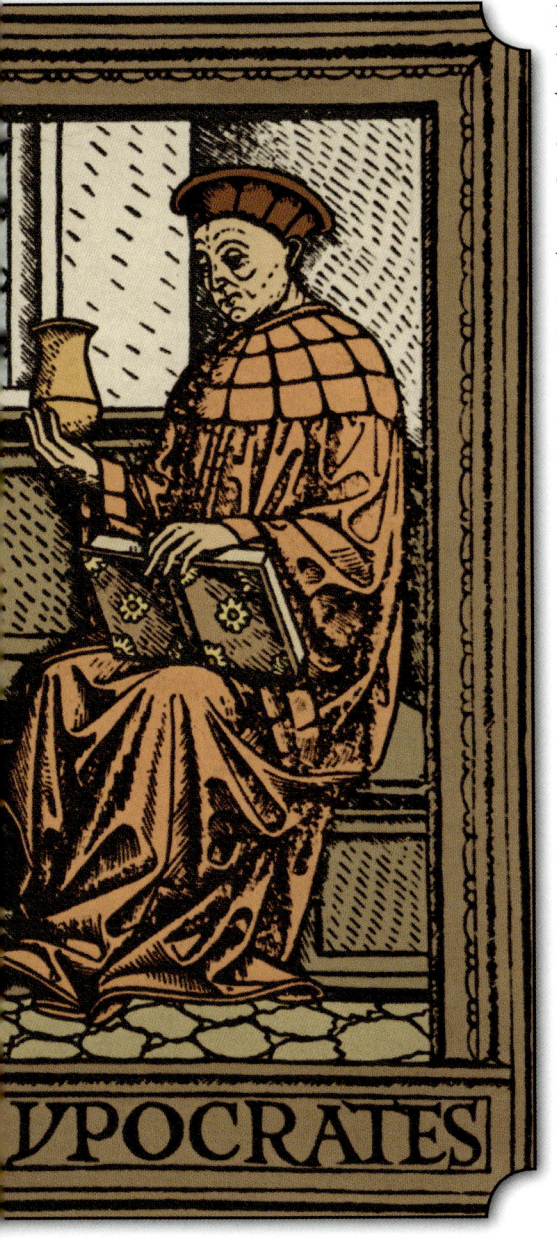

health and built sewers, systems that drained waste water from public baths, and aqueducts that provided clean water.

The ancient Egyptians were among the first to use certain herbs and drugs, including castor oil, senna, and opium. They also set and splinted fractured bones using techniques remarkably similar to those of modern medicine. Egyptians were reputed to be skilled diagnosticians; a medical papyrus from about 1600 BCE, which is believed to be a copy of a text from about 3000 BCE, described 58 sick patients, of whom 42 were given specific diagnoses. Although the Egyptians practiced mummification, which involved removing and dehydrating most of the internal organs of the dead, they apparently did not study those organs, as their anatomical knowledge was quite limited.

Hippocrates (460–375 BCE), known as the "father of Western medicine," was an admired physician and teacher who rejected the notion that disease was punishment sent by the gods; rather, he believed it had natural causes. Hippocrates put forth a doctrine that attributed health and disease to four bodily humours, or fluids—blood, black bile, yellow bile, and phlegm. He believed that the humours were well balanced in a healthy person, but various disturbances or imbalances in them caused disease. At that time, his humoural theory seemed highly scientific. In fact, doctors diagnosed and treated illnesses based on the four humours well into the 19th century.

Knowing that he could not cure most diseases, Hippocrates tended to recommend conservative measures such as exercise, rest, and cleanliness. By contrast, for fever, which he thought was caused by an excess of blood in the body, he recommended the drastic measure of bloodletting. The practice of bloodletting (or bleeding), which was thought to have many therapeutic effects, was used for more than two thousand years and undoubtedly hastened the deaths of countless patients who might otherwise have recovered.

Hippocrates is best known today for his ethical code (Hippocratic Oath), which continues to be used by the medical profession as a guide to appropriate conduct. The oath is a pledge doctors make to always use their knowledge and best judgment for the benefit of patients and to never harm or injure those in their care.

For a brief period after Hippocrates' death, two Greek physician-scholars living in Alexandria, Herophilus and Erasistratus, performed the first known systematic dissections of human bodies. They dissected virtually every organ, including the brain, and recorded what they learned. Despite their dedication to the science of anatomy, these pioneers had little influence on the subsequent practice of medicine. By 150 BCE, dissection of human cadavers was banned throughout the Hellenistic world, and any writings they left behind were lost when Alexandria's library was destroyed in the 3rd century CE.

One of those trained in Hippocratic medicine was Galen (129–216? CE), a Greek who traveled widely and became the most renowned physician in Rome. Although Galen accepted and embellished the four-humours doctrine, he also made important discoveries. He performed systematic experiments on animals (including apes, monkeys, dogs, pigs, snakes, and lions), which involved both dissection and vivisection (live dissection). He treated gladiators and took advantage of the opportunity to study the internal organs and muscles of the wounded. Galen recognized connections between bodily structures and functions; for example, he demonstrated that a severed spinal cord led to paralysis. He recognized that the heart circulated blood through the arteries but did not understand that it circulated in only one direction. Galen produced a prodigious body of medical scholarship that was adhered to by medical practitioners for 1,600 years. Unfortunately, his erroneous beliefs as well as his accurate insights were perpetuated.

After the breakup of the Roman Empire, the tradition of Greek medicine continued in the universities of the Arab world. The Persian physician Rhazes, or al-Rāzī (*c.* 854–925/935), is credited with being the first to distinguish between the highly contagious viral diseases smallpox and measles. He also recognized the need for sanitation in hospitals. Probably the most important physician at the beginning of the second millennium was Avicenna. His monumental *Canon of Medicine*, a five-volume encyclopedia of case histories and therapeutic instructions, was long considered an absolute medical authority in both Eastern and Western traditions.

At about the same time that Arabian medicine flourished, the first medical school in Europe was established at Salerno, in southern Italy. Although the school produced no brilliant genius and no startling discovery, it was the outstanding medical institution of its time. In about 1200 Salerno yielded its place as the premier medical school of Europe to Montpellier, in France. Other great medieval medical schools were founded at Paris, France, and at Bologna and Padua, in Italy.

Even with the presence of these institutions, medicine progressed very slowly in Europe during the Middle Ages. Medieval physicians continued to rely upon ancient medical theories, including that of the humours. They analyzed symptoms, examined waste matter, and made their diagnoses. Then they might prescribe diet, rest, sleep, exercise, or baths, or they could administer emetics (something to cause vomiting) and laxatives or bleed the patient. Surgeons could treat fractures and dislocations, repair hernias, and perform amputations and a few other operations. Some of them prescribed opium or alcohol to deaden pain. Childbirth was left to midwives, who relied on folklore and tradition.

The Christian church also influenced European medicine during the Middle Ages. It is sometimes said that the early church had a negative effect on medical progress. Disease was regarded as a punishment for sin, and healing required only prayer and repentance. A number of saints became associated with miraculous cures of certain diseases, such as St. Vitus for chorea (or St. Vitus's dance) and St. Anthony for erysipelas (or St. Anthony's fire). In addition, the human body was held sacred and dissection was forbidden. Nevertheless, the

— INTRODUCTION —

medieval church played an important role in caring for the sick. Great hospitals were established during the Middle Ages by religious foundations, and infirmaries were attached to abbeys, monasteries, priories, and convents. Doctors and nurses in these institutions were members of religious orders and combined spiritual with physical healing.

It was not until the Renaissance that Europeans began to seek a truly scientific basis for medical knowledge instead of relying on the teachings of Galen and other ancient physicians. The Flemish physician Andreas Vesalius discovered many new principles of anatomy through dissections, which he compiled in his profusely illustrated *De humani corporis fabrica libri septem* ("The Seven Books on the Structure of the Human Body"), published in 1543.

Ambroise Paré (1510–90), a Frenchman, practiced as an army surgeon and became an expert at treating battlefield wounds. He proved that tying blood vessels was a better method of stopping profuse bleeding than cauterizing them with hot oil or a hot iron—a discovery that spared countless soldiers terrible pain and suffering.

Before the mid-1800s surgery had to be performed without anesthesia. Patients may have been given a blow on the head, a dose of opium, or a swig of whiskey or rum—at best, minimally effective means of reducing pain. The best surgeons, therefore, were those who completed their work in the least amount of time. Early in the century British and American scientists began experimenting with two pain-numbing substances, the gas nitrous oxide and the liquid solvent ether. In 1846, before a large group of doctors at Massachusetts General Hospital in Boston, William Morton (who did not have a medical degree but had apprenticed with a dentist) demonstrated ether anesthesia in a patient undergoing surgery to remove a tumor from his neck. The resoundingly successful operation was painless for the patient. Word of this achievement spread quickly, and soon dentists and surgeons on both sides of the Atlantic were using anesthesia. In 1847 chloroform was introduced and became the anesthetic of choice.

Certainly one of the most important advances of the 19th century was the development and acceptance of the "germ theory of disease." In the 1840s Ignaz Semmelweis, a young physician working in a hospital in Vienna, recognized that doctors who performed autopsies and then delivered babies were responsible for spreading puerperal (childbed) fever, an often deadly infection of the reproductive organs. After Semmelweis ordered doctors to wash their hands with a chlorinated lime solution before entering the maternity ward, deaths from puerperal fever plummeted.

French chemist and microbiologist Louis Pasteur first learned about germs by studying the fermentation of beer, wine, and milk. He went on to explore infectious diseases in farm animals and develop vaccines against anthrax in sheep, erysipelas in swine, and chicken cholera in poultry. Finally Pasteur turned his attention to rabies in humans. His crowning achievement was the development of a vaccine against the always-fatal viral infection caused by bites of rabid animals. In 1885 Pasteur was urged by doctors to give his experimental vaccine, which had only been tested in dogs, to a young boy who had been bitten more than a dozen times by a rabid dog. He administered a series of 13 daily injections of increasingly virulent material obtained from the spinal cords of rabid rabbits. The child endured the prolonged and painful treatment and made a full recovery.

German physician Robert Koch discovered that dormant anthrax spores could remain in the blood of sheep for years and, under the right conditions, develop into the infectious organisms that caused deadly anthrax outbreaks. In 1876, when he presented his findings on the anthrax disease cycle to doctors in Breslau, Germany, an eminent pathologist commented: "I regard it as the greatest discovery ever made with bacteria and I believe that this is not the last time that this young Robert Koch will surprise and shame us by the brilliance of his investigations." He was right. Koch went on to discover the bacteria responsible for tuberculosis (TB; 1882) and human cholera (1883) and to do groundbreaking research on leprosy, plague, and malaria.

The French microbiologist Alphonse Laveran discovered the disease-causing protozoan *Plasmodium*, the parasite carried by mosquitoes responsible for malaria. At the turn of the century, the American army doctor Walter Reed headed a team of physicians who proved that yellow fever was also transmitted by mosquitoes.

The first serious studies of mental disease were conducted during the 19th century. Jean Charcot used hypnosis as a tool to search the troubled minds of mental patients. His student Sigmund Freud developed the psychoanalytic technique for treating mental illness.

Throughout the 19th century women in Europe and the United States were actively campaigning for the right to the same education as men, and some notable pioneers succeeded, despite the social obstacles in their way. In 1849 Elizabeth Blackwell, who was born in Britain and whose family immigrated to the United States in 1832, became the first woman to obtain a medical degree. Although the origins of nursing predate the mid-19th century, the history of professional nursing traditionally begins with Florence Nightingale. Nightingale, the well-educated daughter of wealthy British parents, defied social conventions and decided to become a nurse. The work of such women paved the way for numerous others to enter medical professions.

In 1900 the average life expectancy of persons born in the United States was 47 years; by the end of the century it was 77 years. The U.S. Centers for Disease Control and Prevention (CDC) attributed 25 of those 30 additional years of life that Americans had gained to 10 momentous 20th-century public health achievements:

- control of infectious diseases
- immunizations
- the decline in deaths from heart disease and stroke
- safer and healthier foods
- healthier mothers and babies
- increased safety of motor vehicles
- safer workplaces
- family planning
- fluoridation of drinking water
- the recognition of tobacco use as a health hazard

Paul Ehrlich's discovery in 1910 of Salvarsan, the first drug effective against syphilis, inaugurated the era of modern antimicrobial drug therapy. The sulfa drugs, which provided strong protection against streptococci and other bacteria, were introduced in the 1930s. In 1938 Ernst Chain and Howard Florey succeeded in synthesizing and purifying the *Penicillium* mold that Alexander Fleming had discovered 10 years earlier; their product, the broad-spectrum antibiotic penicillin, is still widely used today. In 1948 Selman Waksman discovered streptomycin, a powerful antibiotic that led to the control of tuberculosis (TB).

In the early 1920s researchers Frederick Banting and Charles Best isolated the hormone insulin, which they used to save the lives of young people with diabetes mellitus. At the time, diabetes mainly affected children and adolescents; because their bodies did not produce insulin, which the body needs to convert food into energy, they died. Shortly after this triumph, the pharmaceutical manufacturer Eli Lilly and Company began large-scale production of cow and pig insulin, which helped turn diabetes (the type now known as Type 1) from a fatal into a manageable disease that allowed young people to live into adulthood. By the end of the century, Type 2 diabetes (in which the body is unable to properly utilize the insulin it produces) had become a public health threat of epidemic proportions; 3.8 million people worldwide died from its complications each year.

The eradication of smallpox, one of the most deadly and debilitating scourges the world had ever known, represents one of the greatest accomplishments in modern medicine, science, and public health. Edward Jenner developed the vaccine against smallpox in 1796. Thanks to widespread vaccination, smallpox was eliminated from Europe, North America, Australia, and New Zealand by 1950 and from most of South and Central America by 1959. In 1967 the World Health Organization (WHO) launched a campaign to eradicate the disease that still infected up to 15 million people annually in 31 countries. Ten years later, the last case of smallpox was diagnosed in a young man in Somalia, and in 1980 WHO declared smallpox eradicated from the planet. Because humans were the only natural reservoir of the smallpox virus, once it was gone, people no longer needed to be vaccinated against it. The only remaining specimens of the virus were retained in high-security laboratories in the United States and Russia.

Albert Sabin, building on the work done by Jonas Salk, developed an oral polio vaccine in 1960. A global polio eradication initiative was begun in 1988, at which time about 350,000 children in 125 countries on five continents were crippled each year by the highly contagious viral disease that attacks the nervous system. By 1999 the number of cases had been reduced by 99 percent, and by the end of 2006, only four countries—India, Nigeria, Pakistan, and Afghanistan—still had endemic polio (uninterrupted transmission of the wild polio virus). Continuing efforts reduced the number of cases to just 222 in 2012, and the campaign's sponsors (WHO, the United Nations Children's Fund, CDC, and Rotary International) expressed confidence that a polio-free world could be achieved by 2018.

The early 1980s saw the emergence of the deadly new disease acquired immunodeficiency syndrome (AIDS), caused by the human immunodeficiency virus (HIV), as identified by scientists Luc Montagnier, Francoise Barré-Sinoussi, and Harald zur Hausen in the early 1980s. HIV/AIDS rapidly grew into a global pandemic. Thanks to the development of life-prolonging drugs, by the mid-1990s HIV/AIDS was no longer a death sentence in wealthy countries. In poor countries, however, the pandemic continued to wreak havoc. In 2001 more than 28 million people in sub-Saharan Africa were living with HIV/AIDS, but fewer than 40,000 had access to drug treatment. At the same time, much of Africa and many developing countries were profoundly affected by malaria and TB. The three pandemic diseases killed more than six million people every year.

In 2002 the Global Fund to Fight AIDS, Tuberculosis and Malaria was created to dramatically increase resources to combat the trio of devastating diseases. By mid-2008 the fund had distributed $6.2 billion to 136 countries. At least 1.75 million people were receiving drug treatment for HIV/AIDS, 3.9 million were receiving TB treatment, and 59 million insecticide-treated mosquito nets had been distributed to families in malaria-ridden countries. The program estimated it had saved more than 1.5 million lives.

Late in the 20th century, antimicrobial drugs employed to treat common infections were becoming increasingly ineffective, allowing the return of previously conquered diseases and the emergence of virulent new infections. By 2007 about five percent of the nine million new cases of TB in the world each year were resistant to at least two of the four standard drugs; treatment with other drugs was 200 times more expensive and had lower cure rates. In 2007 the CDC reported that the bacterium methicillin-resistant *Staphylococcus aureus* (MRSA) was responsible for more than 90,000 serious infections and 19,000 deaths in the United States annually. For years MRSA had been a problem in health care institutions such as hospitals, nursing homes, and dialysis centres, where it had grown increasingly resistant to commonly used antibiotics. Formerly it primarily infected people with weakened immune systems; by 2007, however, 13 percent of cases were occurring in healthy people living in the community.

In 1953 British graduate student Francis Crick and American research fellow James Watson drew on the work of British scientist Rosalind Franklin and identified the double-helix structure of deoxyribonucleic acid (DNA), a discovery that helped explain how genetic information is passed along. Exactly 50 years later, the Human Genome Project, led by geneticist Francis Collins, was completed. The 13-year international collaboration of more than 2,800 researchers, one of the boldest scientific undertakings in history, identified all human genes (about 22,000) and determined the sequences of the 3 billion chemical base pairs that make up human DNA. The genetic information provided by the project has enabled researchers to pinpoint errors in genes that cause or contribute to disease. In the future, having the tools to know the precise genetic make-up of individuals will enable clinicians to deliver truly personalized medicine.

    The story of medicine is not just one of diseases, cures, and prevention. Numerous individuals from all walks of life pursuing all manners of interests building on the work of their predecessors have contributed to the advancement of the medical profession. Without the work of the tireless individuals chronicled in the following pages—and the countless others who have dedicated their lives to caring for those in need of medical care—the variety of treatments people enjoy today and the possibilities that continue to be pioneered at the frontiers of medical research could not exist.

IMHOTEP

(born 27th century BCE, Memphis, Egypt–died unknown)

Imhotep (Greek Imouthes) was a vizier, sage, architect, astrologer, and chief minister to Djoser (who reigned 2630–2611 BCE), the second king of Egypt's third dynasty. Imhotep was later worshipped as the god of medicine in Egypt and in Greece, where he was identified with the Greek god of medicine, Asclepius. He is considered to have been the architect of the step pyramid built at the necropolis of Ṣaqqārah in the city of Memphis. The oldest extant monument of hewn stone known to the world, the pyramid consists of six steps and attains a height of 200 feet (61 metres).

Although no contemporary account has been found that refers to Imhotep as a practicing physician, ancient documents illustrating Egyptian society and medicine during the Old Kingdom (c. 2575– c. 2130 BCE) show that the chief magician of the pharaoh's court also frequently served as the nation's chief physician. Imhotep's reputation as the reigning genius of the time, his position in the court, his training as a scribe, and his becoming known as a medical demigod only 100 years after his death are strong indications that he must have been a physician of considerable skill.

Not until the Persian conquest of Egypt in 525 BCE was Imhotep elevated to the position of a full deity, replacing Nefertem in the great triad of Memphis, shared with his mythological parents Ptah, the creator of the universe, and Sekhmet, the goddess of war and pestilence. Imhotep's cult reached its zenith during Greco-Roman times, when his temples in Memphis and on the island of Philae (Arabic: Jazirat Filah) in the Nile River were often crowded with sufferers who prayed and slept there with the

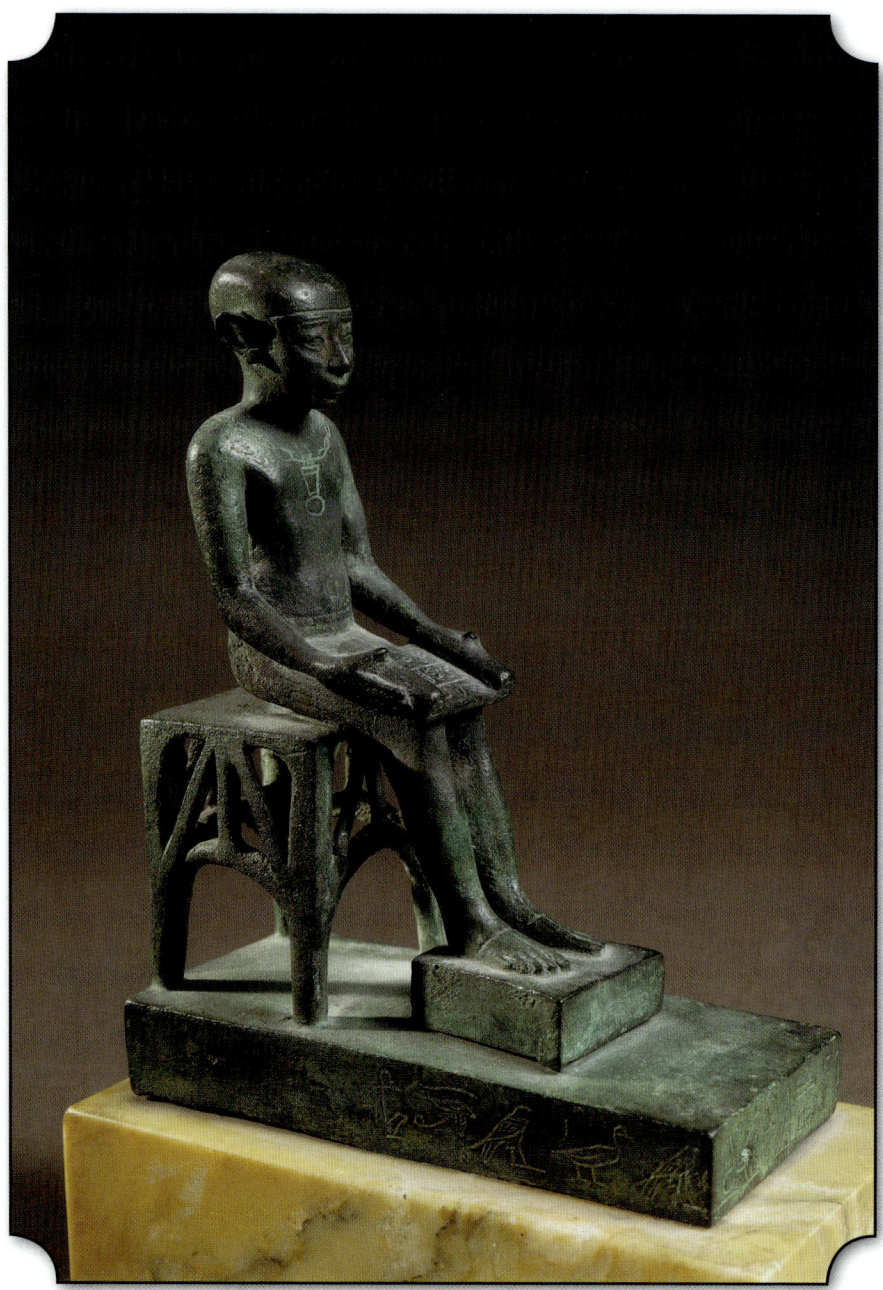

This bronze figure of Imhotep served as an ex-voto, a religious offering in fulfillment of a vow.

conviction that the god would reveal remedies to them in their dreams. The only Egyptian mortal besides the 18th-dynasty sage and minister Amenhotep to attain the honour of total deification, Imhotep is still held in esteem by physicians who, like the eminent 19th-century British practitioner Sir William Osler, consider him "the first figure of a physician to stand out clearly from the mists of antiquity."

HIPPOCRATES

(born *c.* 460 BCE, island of Cos, Greece–died *c.* 375 BCE, Larissa, Thessaly)

Hippocrates was an ancient Greek physician who lived during Greece's Classical period and is traditionally regarded as the father of medicine. It is difficult to isolate the facts of Hippocrates' life from the later tales told about him or to assess his medicine accurately in the face of centuries of reverence for him as the ideal physician. About 60 medical writings have survived that bear his name, most of which were not written by him. He has been revered for his ethical standards in medical practice, mainly for the Hippocratic Oath, which, it is suspected, he did not write.

LIFE AND WORKS

It is known that while Hippocrates was alive, he was admired as a physician and teacher. His younger contemporary Plato referred to him twice. In the *Protagoras* Plato called Hippocrates "the Asclepiad of Cos" who taught students for fees, and he implied that Hippocrates was as well known as a physician as Polyclitus and Phidias were as sculptors. It is now widely accepted that an "Asclepiad" was not a temple priest or a member of a physicians' guild but instead was a physician belonging to a family that had produced well-known physicians for generations. Plato's second reference occurs in the *Phaedrus*, in which Hippocrates is referred to as a famous Asclepiad who had a philosophical approach to medicine.

Meno, a pupil of Aristotle, specifically stated in his history of medicine the views of Hippocrates on the causation of diseases, namely, that undigested residues were produced by unsuitable diet and that these residues excreted vapours, which passed into the body generally and produced diseases. Aristotle said that Hippocrates was called "the Great Physician" but that he was small in stature (*Politics*).

These are the only extant contemporary, or near-contemporary, references to Hippocrates. Five hundred years later, the Greek physician Soranus wrote a life of Hippocrates, but the contents of this and later lives were largely traditional or imaginative. Throughout his life Hippocrates appears to have traveled widely in Greece and Asia Minor practicing his art and teaching his pupils, and he presumably taught at the medical school at Cos quite frequently. His birth and death dates are traditional but may well be approximately accurate. Undoubtedly, Hippocrates was a historical figure, a great physician who exercised a permanent influence on the development of medicine and on the ideals and ethics of the physician.

Hippocrates' reputation, and myths about his life and his family, began to grow in the Hellenistic period, about a century after his death. During this period, the Museum of Alexandria in Egypt collected for its library literary material from preceding periods in celebration of the past greatness of Greece. So far as it can be inferred, the medical works that remained from the Classical period (among the earliest prose writings in Greek) were assembled as a group and called the works of Hippocrates (*Corpus*

Hippocraticum). Linguists and physicians subsequently wrote commentaries on them, and, as a result, all the virtues of the Classical medical works were eventually attributed to Hippocrates and his personality constructed from them.

The virtues of the Hippocratic writings are many, and, although they are of varying lengths and literary quality, they are all simple and direct, earnest in their desire to help, and lacking in technical jargon and elaborate argument. The works show such different views and styles that they cannot be by one person, and some were clearly written in later periods. Yet all the works of the *Corpus* share basic assumptions about how the body works and what disease is, providing a sense of the substance and appeal of ancient Greek medicine as practiced by Hippocrates and other physicians of his era. Prominent among these attractive works are the *Epidemics*, which give annual records of weather and associated diseases, along with individual case histories and records of treatment, collected from cities in northern Greece. Diagnosis and prognosis are frequent subjects. Other treatises explain how to set fractures and treat wounds, feed and comfort patients, and take care of the body to avoid illness. Treatises called *Diseases* deal with serious illnesses, proceeding from the head to the feet, giving symptoms, prognoses, and treatments. There are works on diseases of women, childbirth, and pediatrics. Prescribed medications, other than foods and local salves, are generally purgatives to rid the body of the noxious substances thought to cause disease. Some works argue that medicine is indeed a science, with firm principles and methods, although explicit medical theory is very rare. The medicine depends on a mythology of how the body works and how its inner organs are connected. The myth is laboriously constructed from experience, but it must be remembered that there was neither systematic research nor dissection of human beings in Hippocrates' time. Hence, while much of the writing seems wise and correct, there are large areas where much is unknown.

The Embassy, a fictional work that connects Hippocrates' family with critical events in the history of Cos and Greece, was included in the original collection of Hippocratic works in the Library of Alexandria. Over the next four centuries, *The Embassy* inspired other imaginative writings, including letters between Hippocrates and the Persian king and also the philosopher Democritus. Though obviously fiction, these works enhanced Hippocrates' reputation, providing the basis for later biographies and the traditional picture of Hippocrates as the father of medicine. Still other works were added to the Hippocratic *Corpus* between its first collection and its first scholarly edition around the beginning of the 2nd century CE. Among them were the Hippocratic Oath and other ethical writings that prescribe principles of behaviour for the physician.

Hippocratic Oath

The Hippocratic Oath is an ethical code attributed to Hippocrates. It was adopted as a guide to conduct by the medical profession throughout the ages and still used in the graduation ceremonies of many medical schools. In addition to containing information on medical matters, the *Corpus* embodied a code of principles for the teachers of medicine and for their students. This code, or a fragment of it, has been handed down in various versions through generations of physicians as the Hippocratic oath.

The oath dictates the obligations of the physician to students of medicine and the duties of pupil to teacher. In the oath, the physician pledges to prescribe only beneficial treatments, according to his abilities and judgment; to refrain from causing harm or hurt; and to live an exemplary personal and professional life.

The text of the Hippocratic Oath (*c.* 400 BCE) provided below is a translation from Greek by Francis Adams (1849). It is considered a classical version and differs from contemporary versions, which are reviewed and revised frequently to fit with changes in modern medical practice.

> I swear by Apollo the physician, and Aesculapius, and Health, and All-heal, and all the gods and goddesses, that, according to my ability and judgment, I will keep this Oath and this stipulation—to reckon him who taught me this Art equally dear to me as my parents, to share my substance with him, and relieve his necessities if required; to look upon his offspring in the same footing as my own brothers, and to teach them this Art, if they shall wish to learn it, without fee or stipulation; and that by precept, lecture, and every other mode of instruction, I will impart a knowledge of the Art to my own sons, and those of my teachers, and to disciples bound by a stipulation and oath according to the law of medicine, but to none others. I will follow that system of regimen which, according to my ability and judgment, I consider for the benefit of my patients, and abstain from whatever is deleterious and mischievous. I will give no deadly medicine to any one if asked, nor suggest any such counsel; and in like manner I will not give to a woman a pessary to produce abortion. With purity and with holiness I will pass my life and practice my Art. I will not cut persons laboring under the stone, but will leave this to be done by men who are

practitioners of this work. Into whatever houses I enter, I will go into them for the benefit of the sick, and will abstain from every voluntary act of mischief and corruption; and, further from the seduction of females or males, of freemen and slaves. Whatever, in connection with my professional practice or not, in connection with it, I see or hear, in the life of men, which ought not to be spoken of abroad, I will not divulge, as reckoning that all such should be kept secret. While I continue to keep this Oath unviolated, may it be granted to me to enjoy life and the practice of the art, respected by all men, in all times! But should I trespass and violate this Oath, may the reverse be my lot!

INFLUENCE

Technical medical science developed in the Hellenistic period and after. Surgery, pharmacy, and anatomy advanced; physiology became the subject of serious speculation; and philosophic criticism improved the logic of medical theories. Competing schools in medicine (first Empiricism and later Rationalism) claimed Hippocrates as the origin and inspiration of their doctrines. In the 2nd century CE, the physician Galen of Pergamum developed his magnificent medical system, a synthesis of preceding work and his own additions that became the basis of European and Arabic medicine into the Renaissance. Galen was argumentative and long-winded, often abusive of contemporaries and earlier physicians, but at the same time, with exaggerated reverence that ignored five centuries of progress, he claimed that Hippocrates was the source of all that he himself knew and practiced. For later physicians, Hippocrates stood as the inspirational source, while the more difficult Galen offered the substantial details.

As time went on, reverence for the past had to contend with new notions of scientific method and new discoveries. In the process, Galen's authority was undone, but Hippocrates' eminence as father of medicine remained. Scientific progress in fields such as anatomy, chemistry, microbiology, and microscopy, especially beginning in the 16th and 17th centuries, demanded that Galen's medicine be criticized and revised part by part. Arguments against Galenic medicine were often more effective when they were presented as returns to true Hippocratic medicine. New scientific methodology argued for a return to observation and study of nature, abandoning bookish authority. The simple and direct writings of the Hippocratic Collection read well as sample empirical texts that eschewed dogma. By the late 19th century, Galen was irrelevant to medical practice, and general knowledge of Hippocratic medical writings was beginning to fade. However, today Hippocrates still continues to represent the humane, ethical aspects of the medical profession.

A number of idealized images of Hippocrates have survived from antiquity, but none that seems to derive from a contemporary portrait.

PEDANIUS DIOSCORIDES
(born *c.* 40 CE, Anazarbus, Cilicia–died *c.* 90)

Pedanius Dioscorides was a Greek physician and pharmacologist whose work *De materia medica* was the foremost classical source of modern botanical terminology and the leading pharmacological text for 16 centuries.

Dioscorides' travels as a surgeon with the armies of the Roman emperor Nero provided him an opportunity to study the features, distribution, and medicinal properties of many plants and minerals. Excellent descriptions of nearly 600 plants, including cannabis, colchicum, water hemlock, and peppermint, are contained in *De materia medica*. Written in five books around the year 77, this work deals with approximately 1,000 simple drugs.

The medicinal and dietetic value of animal derivatives such as milk and honey is described in the second book, and a synopsis of such chemical drugs as mercury (with directions for its preparation from cinnabar), arsenic (referred to as auripigmentum, the yellow arsenic sulfide), lead acetate, calcium hydrate, and copper oxide is found in the fifth book. He clearly refers to sleeping potions prepared from opium and mandragora as surgical anesthetics.

Although the work may be considered little more than a drug collector's manual by modern standards, the original Greek manuscript, which was copied in at least seven other languages, describes most drugs used in medical practice until modern times and served as the primary text of pharmacology until the end of the 15th century. Modern editions have been published in Greek (1906–14) and in English (1934).

GALEN OF PERGAMUM
(born 129 CE, Pergamum, Mysia, Anatolia [now Bergama, Turkey]–died *c.* 216)

Galen of Pergamum was a Greek physician, writer, and philosopher who exercised a dominant influence on medical theory and practice in Europe from the Middle Ages until the mid-17th century. His authority in the Byzantine world and the Muslim Middle East was similarly long-lived.

Early Life and Training

The son of a wealthy architect, Galen was educated as a philosopher and man of letters. His hometown, Pergamum, was the site of a magnificent shrine of the healing god, Asclepius, that was visited by many distinguished figures of the Roman Empire for cures. When Galen was 16, he changed his career to that of medicine, which he studied at Pergamum, at Smyrna (modern Izmir, Turkey), and finally at Alexandria in Egypt, which was the greatest medical centre of the ancient world. After more than a decade of study, he returned in 157 CE to Pergamum, where he served as chief physician to the troop of gladiators maintained by the high priest of Asia.

In 162 the ambitious Galen moved to Rome. There he quickly rose in the medical profession owing to his public

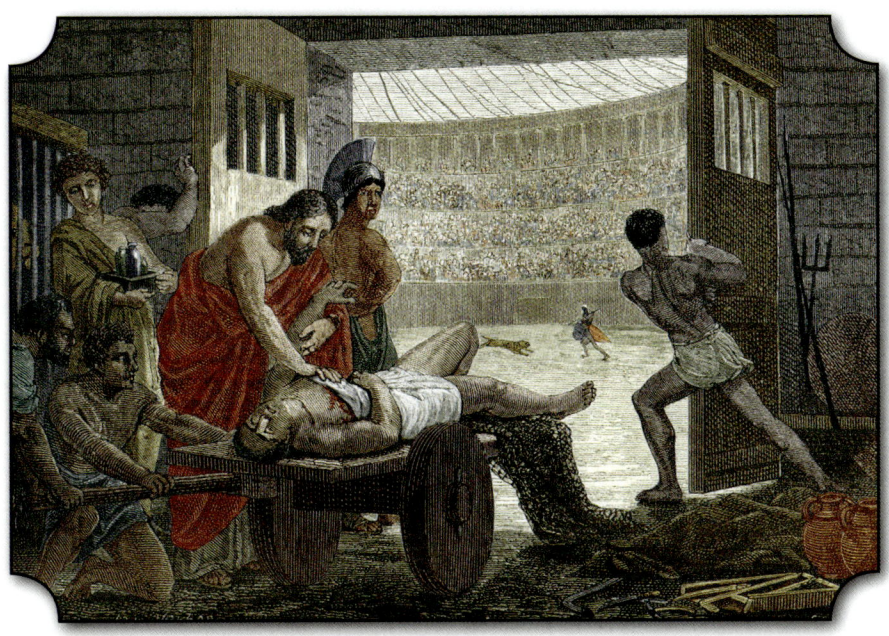

In this rendering, Galen treats a wounded gladiator in Pergamum, his place of birth.

demonstrations of anatomy, his successes with rich and influential patients whom other doctors had pronounced incurable, his enormous learning, and the rhetorical skills he displayed in public debates. Galen's wealthy background, social contacts, and a friendship with his old philosophy teacher Eudemus further enhanced his reputation as a philosopher and physician.

Galen abruptly ended his sojourn in the capital in 166. Although he claimed that the intolerable envy of his colleagues prompted his return to Pergamum, an impending plague in Rome was probably a more compelling reason. In 168–169, however, he was called by the joint emperors Lucius Verus and Marcus Aurelius to accompany them on a military campaign in northern Italy. After Verus's sudden death in 169, Galen returned to Rome, where he served Marcus Aurelius and the later emperors Commodus and Septimius Severus as a physician. Galen's final works were written after 207, which suggests that his Arab biographers were correct in their claim that he died at age 87, in 216/217.

Anatomical and Medical Studies

Galen regarded anatomy as the foundation of medical knowledge, and he frequently dissected and experimented on such lower animals as the Barbary ape (or African monkey), pigs, sheep, and goats. Galen's advocacy of dissection, both to improve surgical skills and for research purposes, formed part of his self-promotion, but there is no doubt that he was an accurate observer. He distinguished seven pairs of cranial nerves, described the valves of the heart, and observed the structural differences between arteries and veins. One of his most important demonstrations was that the arteries carry blood, not air, as had been taught for 400 years. Notable also were his vivisection experiments, which involved performing experiments on live animals. These experiments included tying off the recurrent laryngeal nerve (a nerve supplying the larynx) to show that the brain controls the voice; performing a series of transections of the spinal cord to establish the functions of the spinal nerves; and tying off the ureters (ducts between the kidney and bladder or cloaca) to demonstrate kidney and bladder functions. Galen was seriously hampered by the prevailing social taboo against dissecting human corpses, however, and the inferences he made about human anatomy based on his dissections of animals often led him into errors. His anatomy of the uterus, for example, is largely that of the dog's.

Galen's physiology was a mixture of ideas taken from the philosophers Plato and Aristotle as well as from the physician Hippocrates, whom Galen revered as the fount of all medical learning. Galen viewed the body as consisting of three connected systems: the brain and nerves, which are responsible for sensation and thought; the heart and arteries, responsible for life-giving energy; and the liver and veins, responsible for nutrition and growth. According to Galen, blood is formed in the liver and is then carried by the veins to all parts of the body, where it is used up as nutriment or is transformed into flesh and other substances. A small amount of blood seeps through the lungs between the pulmonary artery and pulmonary veins, thereby becoming mixed with air, and then seeps from the right to the left ventricle of the heart through minute pores in the wall separating the two chambers. A small proportion of this blood is further refined in a network of nerves at the base of the skull (in reality found only in ungulates) and the brain to make psychic pneuma, a subtle material that is the vehicle of sensation. Galen's physiological theory proved extremely seductive, and few possessed the skills needed to challenge it in succeeding centuries.

Building on earlier Hippocratic conceptions, Galen believed that human health requires an equilibrium between the four main bodily fluids, or humours—blood, yellow bile, black bile, and phlegm. Each of the humours is built up from the four elements and displays two of the four primary qualities: hot, cold, wet, and dry. Unlike Hippocrates, Galen argued that humoural imbalances can be located in specific organs, as well as in the body as a whole. This modification of the theory allowed doctors to make more precise diagnoses and to prescribe specific remedies to restore the body's balance. As a continuation of earlier Hippocratic conceptions, Galenic physiology became a powerful influence in medicine for the next 1,400 years.

Galen was both a universal genius and a prolific writer: about 300 titles of works by him are known, of which about 150 survive wholly or in part. He was perpetually inquisitive, even in areas remote from medicine, such as linguistics, and he was an important logician who wrote major studies of scientific method. Galen was also a skilled polemicist and an incorrigible publicist of his own genius, and these traits, combined with the enormous range of his writings, help to explain his subsequent fame and influence.

INFLUENCE

Galen's writings achieved wide circulation during his lifetime, and copies of some of his works survive that were written within a generation of his death. By 500 CE his works were being taught and summarized at Alexandria, and his theories were already crowding out those of others in the medical handbooks of the Byzantine world. Greek manuscripts began to be collected and translated by enlightened Arabs in the 9th century, and about 850

Ḥunayn ibn Isḥāq, an Arab physician at the court of Baghdad, prepared an annotated list of 129 works of Galen that he and his followers had translated from Greek into Arabic or Syriac. Learned medicine in the Arabic world thus became heavily based upon the commentary, exposition, and understanding of Galen.

Galen's influence was initially almost negligible in western Europe except for drug recipes, but from the late 11th century Ḥunayn's translations, commentaries on them by Arab physicians, and sometimes the original Greek writings themselves were translated into Latin. These Latin versions came to form the basis of medical education in the new medieval universities. From about 1490, Italian humanists felt the need to prepare new Latin versions of Galen directly from Greek manuscripts in order to free his texts from medieval preconceptions and misunderstandings. Galen's works were first printed in Greek in their entirety in 1525, and printings in Latin swiftly followed. These texts offered a different picture from that of the Middle Ages, one that emphasized Galen as a clinician, a diagnostician, and above all, an anatomist. His new followers stressed his methodical techniques of identifying and curing illness, his independent judgment, and his cautious empiricism. Galen's injunctions to investigate the body were eagerly followed, since physicians wished to repeat the experiments and observations that he had recorded. Paradoxically, this soon led to the overthrow of Galen's authority as an anatomist. In 1543 the Flemish physician Andreas Vesalius showed that Galen's anatomy of the body was more animal than human in some of its aspects, and it became clear that Galen and his medieval followers had made many errors. Galen's notions of physiology, by contrast, lasted for a further century, until the English physician William Harvey correctly explained the circulation of the blood. The renewal and then the overthrow of the Galenic tradition in the Renaissance had been an important element in the rise of modern science, however.

HUA TUO
(flourished *c.* late 2nd century CE–early 3rd century)

Hua Tuo was a Chinese physician and surgeon who is best known for his surgical operations and the use of mafeisan, an herbal anesthetic formulation made from hemp.

Ancient Chinese doctors felt that surgery was a matter of last resort, and little time was spent teaching or describing surgical techniques. What surgery was done was usually carried out by a lower grade of medical worker. However, around the beginning of the 3rd century Hua Tuo began to change Chinese surgery. As a young man, Hua Tuo traveled and read widely. He probably first became interested in medicine while trying to help the countless soldiers who had been wounded in the many wars of that violent period.

As a young surgeon, Hua Tuo believed in simplicity, using only a few prescriptions and a few points for acupuncture. Using a preparation of hemp and wine, he was able to make his patients insensitive to pain. Hua Tuo is believed by some to have been the discoverer of anesthetics, although it is possible that the Chinese physician Bian Qiao, who lived in the 5th century BCE, had used them. Hua Tuo engaged in a wide variety of surgical procedures including laparotomy (incision into the abdominal cavity), removal of diseased tissues, and even a partial splenectomy (removal of the spleen). To treat gastrointestinal diseases Hua Tuo's favourite procedure was to resect the viscera and wash the inside. He probably even performed end-to-end anastomoses (connections) of the intestines, although it is not known what substance he used for the sutures.

Of the stories told of Hua Tuo, one—possibly fabricated—is that General Guan Di (Kuan Ti), one of the great military heroes of the time who eventually became the god of war, came to Hua Tuo because of an arrow wound in his arm that had become badly infected. The surgeon prepared to give his patient the usual anesthetic drink, but General Guandi laughed scornfully and called for a board and stones for a game of go. While Hua Tuo scraped the flesh and bone free of infection and repaired the wound, Guandi and one of his military companions proceeded calmly with their game.

Surgery, although his main interest, was only one of Hua Tuo's pursuits. He pioneered in hydrotherapy, and he did innovative work in physiotherapy. His series of exercises known as the frolics of the five animals, in which the patient imitated movements of the tiger, deer, bear, ape, and bird, was well known and widely adopted.

The end of Hua Tuo's life is hidden in a mist of conflicting and doubtful stories. A likely set of these has him late in life becoming court physician to Cao Cao, king of Wei. The surgeon temporarily relieved the ruler of his giddiness by acupuncture. When the king asked him to do something to remove this annoyance permanently, Hua Tuo said he would have to cut into the royal skull. Cao Cao's wife was in favour of surgery as a desperate hope, but the king became suspicious that his enemies had bribed Hua Tuo to kill him. In a fit of rage, perhaps triggered by his headaches, the king had the surgeon thrown into jail and executed. Hua Tuo's major book, *Qingnangshu* (*Book of the Blue Bag*) was burned, either by the jailer who wanted to remove all traces of the prisoner or by the surgeon's wife acting in accordance with Hua Tuo's wishes expressed before he was jailed.

Hua Tuo earned his place as the greatest surgeon in Chinese history. Unfortunately, the destruction of his writings and the Confucian dogma against mutilation of the human body combined to prevent the growth of surgery that might have been expected to follow the life of such a remarkable pioneer.

AL-RĀZĪ

(born *c.* 854, Rayy, Persia [now in Iran]–died 925/935, Rayy)

Al-Rāzī (in full, Abū Bakr Muḥammad ibn Zakariyyā' al-Rāzī) was a celebrated alchemist and Muslim philosopher who is also considered to have been the greatest physician of the Islamic world. One tradition holds that al-Rāzī was already an alchemist before he gained his medical knowledge. After serving as chief physician in a Rayy hospital, he held a similar position in Baghdad for some time. Like many intellectuals in his day, he lived at various small courts under the patronage of minor rulers. With references to his Greek predecessors, al-Rāzī viewed himself as the Islamic version of Socrates in philosophy and of Hippocrates in medicine.

Al-Rāzī's two most significant medical works are the *Kitāb al-Manṣūrī*, which he composed for the Rayy ruler Manṣūr ibn Isḥaq and which became well known in the West in Gerard of Cremona's 12th-century Latin translation; and *Kitāb al-ḥāwī*, the "Comprehensive Book," in which he surveyed Greek, Syrian, and early Arabic medicine, as well as some Indian medical knowledge. Throughout his works he added his own considered judgment and his own medical experience as commentary.

Among his numerous minor medical treatises is the famed *Treatise on the Small Pox and Measles*, which was translated into Latin, Byzantine Greek, and various modern languages.

The philosophical writings of al-Rāzī were neglected for centuries, and renewed appreciation of their importance did not occur until the 20th century. Although he claimed to be a follower of Plato, he consistently disagreed with such Arabic interpreters of Plato as al-Fārābī, Avicenna (Ibn Sīnā), and Averroës (Ibn Rushd). He was probably acquainted with Arabic translations of the Greek atomist philosopher Democritus and pursued a similar tendency in his own atomic theory of the composition of matter. Among his other works, *The Spiritual Physick of Rhazes* is a popular ethical treatise and a major alchemical study.

AVICENNA

(born 980, near Bukhara, Iran [now in Uzbekistan]–died 1037, Hamadan, Iran)

Avicenna (in full Abū ʿAlī al-Ḥusayn ibn ʿAbd Allāh ibn Sīnā) was a Muslim physician and the most famous and influential of the philosopher-scientists of the medieval Islamic world. He was particularly noted for his contributions in the fields of Aristotelian philosophy and medicine. He composed the *Kitāb al-shifāʾ* (*Book of the Cure*), a vast philosophical and scientific encyclopaedia, and *Al-Qānūn fī al-ṭibb* (*The Canon of Medicine*), which is among the most famous books in the history of medicine.

Avicenna did not burst upon an empty Islamic intellectual stage. It is believed that Muslim writer Ibn al-Muqaffaʿ, or possibly his son, had introduced

Aristotelian logic to the Islamic world more than two centuries before Avicenna. Al-Kindī, the first Islamic Peripatetic (Aristotelian) philosopher, and Turkish polymath al-Fārābī, from whose book Avicenna would learn Aristotle's metaphysics, preceded him. Of these luminaries, however, Avicenna remains by far the greatest.

LIFE AND EDUCATION

According to Avicenna's personal account of his life, as communicated in the records of his longtime pupil al-Jūzjānī, he read and memorized the entire Qurʾān by age 10. The tutor Nātilī instructed the youth in elementary logic, and, having soon surpassed his teacher, Avicenna took to studying the Hellenistic authors on his own. By age 16 Avicenna turned to medicine, a discipline over which he claimed "easy" mastery. When the sultan of Bukhara fell ill with an ailment that baffled the court physicians, Avicenna was called to his bedside and cured him. In gratitude, the sultan opened the royal Sāmānid library to him, a fortuitous benevolence that introduced Avicenna to a veritable cornucopia of science and philosophy.

Avicenna began his prodigious writing career at age 21. Some 240 extant titles bear his name. They cross numerous fields, including mathematics, geometry, astronomy, physics, metaphysics, philology, music, and poetry. Often caught up in the tempestuous political and religious strife of the era, Avicenna's scholarship was unquestionably hampered by a need to remain on the move. At Eṣfahān, under ʿAlā al-Dawla, he found the stability and security that had eluded him. If Avicenna could be said to have had any halcyon days, they occurred during his time at Eṣfahān, where he was insulated from political intrigues and could hold his own scholars' court every Friday, discussing topics at will. In this salubrious climate, Avicenna completed *Kitāb al-shifā'*, wrote *Dānish nāma-i 'alā'ī* (*Book of Knowledge*) and *Kitāb al-najāt* (*Book of Salvation*), and compiled new and more-accurate astronomical tables.

While in the company of 'Alā al-Dawla, Avicenna fell ill with colic. He treated himself by employing the heroic measure of eight self-administered celery-seed enemas in one day. However, the preparation was either inadvertently or intentionally altered by an attendant to include five measures of active ingredient instead of the prescribed two. That caused ulceration of the intestines. Following up with mithridate (a mild opium remedy attributed to Mithradates VI Eupator, king of Pontus [120–63 BCE]), a slave attempted to poison Avicenna by surreptitiously adding a surfeit of opium. Weakened but indefatigable, he accompanied 'Alā al-Dawla on his march to Hamadan. On the way he took a severe turn for the worse, lingered for a while, and died in the holy month of Ramadan.

INFLUENCE IN PHILOSOPHY AND SCIENCE

In 1919–20 British Orientalist and acclaimed authority on Persia Edward G. Browne opined that "Avicenna was a better philosopher than physician, but al-Rāzī [Rhazes] a better physician than philosopher," a conclusion oft repeated ever since. But a judgment issued 800 years later begs the question: By what contemporary measure is an appraisal of "better" made? Several points are needed to make the philosophical and scientific views of these men comprehensible today. Theirs was the culture of the 'Abbāsid Caliphate (750–1258), the final ruling dynasty built on the precepts of the first Muslim community (*ummah*) in the Islamic world. Thus, their cultural beliefs were remote from those of the 20th-century West and those of their Hellenistic predecessors. Their worldview was theocentric (centred on God)—rather than anthropocentric (centred on humans), a perspective known to the Greco-Roman world. Their cosmology was a unity of natural, supernatural, and preternatural realms.

Avicenna's cosmology centralized God as the Creator—the First Cause, the necessary Being from whom emanated the 10 intelligences and whose immutable essence and existence reigned over those intelligences. The First Intelligence descended on down to the Active Intelligence, which communicated to humans through its divine light, a symbolic attribute deriving authority from the Qurʾān.

Avicenna's most important work of philosophy and science is *Kitāb al-shifāʾ*, which is a four-part encyclopaedia covering logic, physics, mathematics, and metaphysics. Since science was equated with wisdom, Avicenna attempted a broad unified classification of knowledge. For example, in the physics section, nature is discussed in the context of eight principal sciences, including the sciences of general principles, of celestial and terrestrial bodies, and of primary elements, as well as meteorology, mineralogy, botany, zoology, and psychology (science of the soul). The subordinate sciences, in order of importance, as designated by Avicenna, are medicine; astrology; physiognomy, the study of the correspondence of psychological characteristics to physical structure; oneiromancy, the art of dream interpretation; talismans, objects with magical power to blend the celestial forces with the forces of particular worldly bodies, giving rise to extraordinary action on earth; theurgy, the "secrets of prodigies," whereby the combining of terrestrial forces are made to produce remarkable actions and effects; and alchemy, an arcane art studied by Avicenna, although he ultimately rejected its transmutationism (the notion that base metals, such as copper and lead, could be transformed into precious metals, such as gold and silver). Mathematics is divided into four principal sciences: numbers and arithmetic, geometry and geography, astronomy, and music.

Logic was viewed by Avicenna as instrumental to philosophy, an art and a science to be concerned with second-order concepts. While he was generally within the tradition of al-Fārābī and al-Kindī, he more clearly dissociated himself from the Peripatetic school of Baghdad and utilized concepts of the Platonic and Stoic doctrines more openly and with a more independent mind. More importantly, his theology—the First Cause and the 10 intelligences—allowed his philosophy, with its devotion to God as Creator and the celestial hierarchy, to be imported easily into medieval European Scholastic thought.

Influence in Medicine

Despite a general assessment favouring al-Rāzī's medical contributions, many physicians historically preferred Avicenna for his organization and clarity. Indeed, his influence over Europe's great medical schools extended well into the early modern period. There *The Canon of Medicine* (*Al-Qānūn fī al-ṭibb*) became the preeminent source, rather than al-Rāzī's *Kitāb al-ḥāwī* (*Comprehensive Book*).

Avicenna's penchant for categorizing becomes immediately evident in the *Canon*, which is divided into five books. The first book contains four treatises, the first of

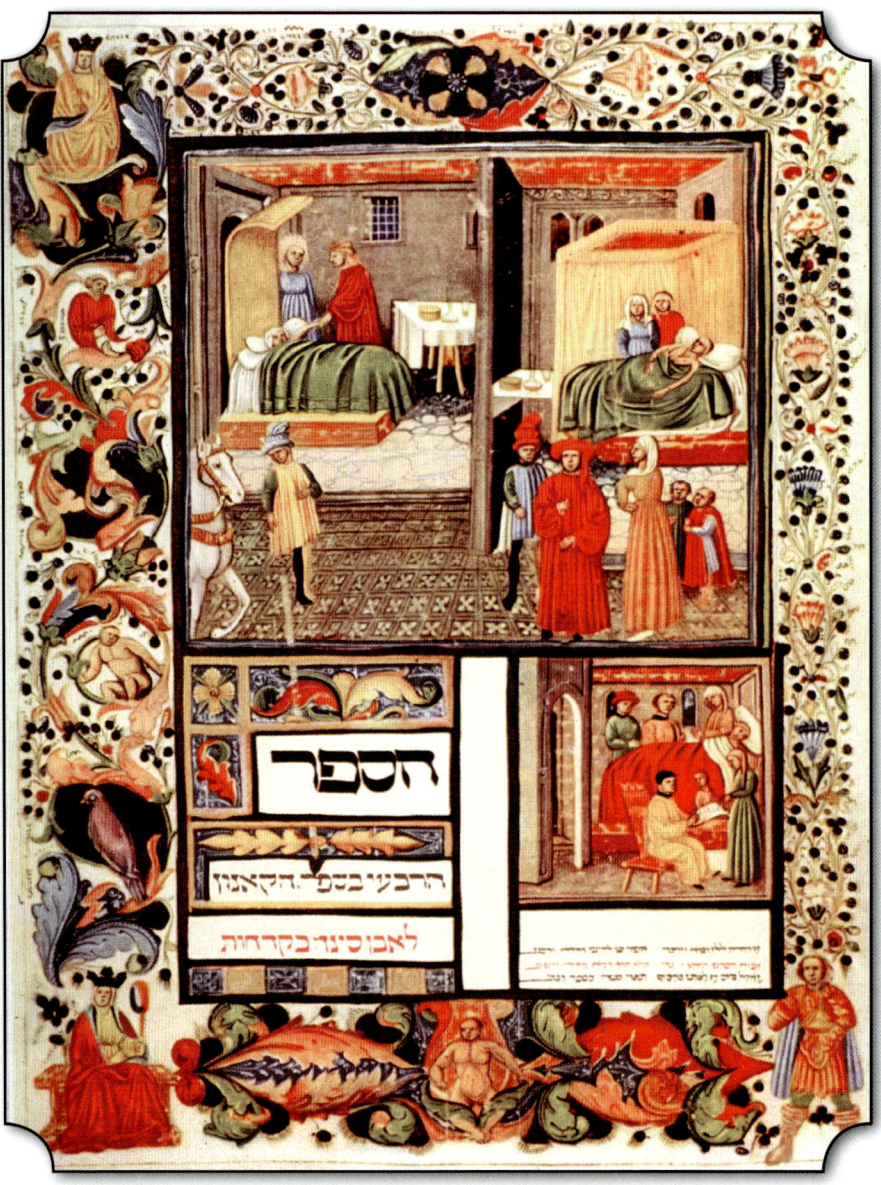

This 15th-century miniature from Avicenna's Canon *depicts the three stages of a medical visit from a physician: examination, consultation, and prescription.*

which examines the four elements (earth, air, fire, and water) in light of Greek physician Galen of Pergamum's four humours (blood, phlegm, yellow bile, and black bile). The first treatise also includes anatomy. The second treatise examines etiology (cause) and symptoms, while the third covers hygiene, health and sickness, and death's inevitability. The fourth treatise is a therapeutic nosology (classification of disease) and a general overview of regimens and dietary treatments. Book II of the *Canon* is a "Materia Medica," Book III covers "Head-to-Toe Diseases," Book IV examines "Diseases That Are Not Specific to Certain Organs" (fevers and other systemic and humoural pathologies), and Book V presents "Compound Drugs" (e.g., theriacs, mithridates, electuaries, and cathartics—antidotes to poison and other medications). Books II and V each offer important compendia of about 760 simple and compound drugs that elaborate upon Galen's humoural pathology.

Unfortunately, Avicenna's original clinical records, intended as an appendix to the *Canon*, were lost, and only an Arabic text has survived in a Roman publication of 1593. Yet, he obviously practiced Greek physician Hippocrates' treatment of spinal deformities with reduction techniques, an approach that had been refined by Greek physician and surgeon Paul of Aegina. Reduction involved the use of pressure and traction to straighten or otherwise correct bone and joint deformities such as curvature of the spine. The techniques were not used again until French surgeon Jean-François Calot reintroduced the practice in 1896. Avicenna's suggestion of wine as a wound dressing was commonly employed in medieval Europe. He also described a condition known as "Persian fire" (anthrax), correctly correlated the sweet taste of urine to diabetes, and described the guinea worm.

Avicenna's influence extends into modern medical practice. Evidence-based medicine, for example, is often presented as a wholly contemporary phenomenon driven by the double-blind clinical trial. But, as medical historian Michael McVaugh pointed out, medieval physicians went to great pains to build their practices upon reliable evidence. Here, Avicenna played a leading role as a prominent figure within the Greco-Arabic literature that influenced such 13th-century physicians as Arnold of Villanova (c. 1235–1313), Bernard de Gordon (fl. 1270–1330), and Nicholas of Poland (c. 1235–1316). It was Avicenna's concept of a *proprietas* (a consistently effective remedy founded directly upon experience) that permitted the testing and confirmation of remedies within a context of rational causation. Avicenna, and to a lesser extent Rhazes, gave many prominent medieval healers a framework of medicine as an empirical science integral to what McVaugh called "a rational schema of nature." This should not be assumed to have led medieval physicians to construct a modern nosology or to develop modern research protocols. However, it is equally ahistorical to dismiss the contributions of Avicenna, and the Greco-Arabic literature of which he was such a prominent part, to the construction of modalities of care that were fundamentally evidence-based.

Assessment

It is difficult to fully assess Avicenna's personal life. Most of what is known of Avicenna is found in the autobiography dictated to his longtime protégé al-Jūzjānī. While his life was embellished by friends and vilified by foes, by all accounts he loved life and had a voracious appetite for lively music, strong drink, and promiscuity. Avicenna's mercurial wit and expansive brilliance won him many friends, but his flaunting of Islamic puritanical conventions earned him even more enemies. At times he appears arrogant. While he borrowed heavily from al-Rāzī, Avicenna dismissed his Persian predecessor by insisting that he should have stuck "to testing stools and urine." Avicenna also appears to have been a lonely, brooding figure, whose efforts at self-promotion were often tempered by a cagey instinct for survival in a politically volatile world. Despite Avicenna's personal strengths and weaknesses, his intelligence was great in theoretical and practical matters.

In addition to Avicenna's philosophy having been readily incorporated into medieval European Scholastic thought, his synthesis of Neoplatonic and Aristotelian thought and his encompassing of all human knowledge of the time into well-organized accessible texts make him one of the greatest intellects since Aristotle. British philosopher Antony Flew's appraisal of Avicenna as "one of the greatest thinkers ever to write in Arabic" expresses the modern scholarly assessment of the man.

In medicine, Avicenna exerted a profound influence over the schools of Europe into the 17th century. The *Canon* was subjected to increasing criticism by Renaissance instructors, yet, because Avicenna's text adhered to the practice and theories of medicine described in Greco-Roman texts, instructors used it to introduce their students to the basic principles of science. Avicenna, never wanting for enemies, was as true in death as in life. Medieval physician Arnold of Villanova berated Avicenna as "a professional scribbler who had stupefied European physicians by his misinterpretation of Galen." But such an assertion is heavy-handed. Indeed, without Avicenna much knowledge would have been lost. Furthermore, his resilience over the centuries belies Villanova's conclusion. Lecturing in 1913, Canadian physician and professor of medicine Sir William Osler described Avicenna as "the author of the most famous medical text-book ever written." Osler added that Avicenna, as a practitioner, was "the prototype of the successful physician who was at the same time statesman, teacher, philosopher and literary man."

Taken in his entirety, Avicenna must be seen in context with his Islamic colleagues—al-Rāzī, Ibn Rushd (Averroës), ʿAlī ibn al-ʿAbbās (Haly Abbas), Abū al-Qāsim (Albucasis), Ibn Zuhr (Avenzoar), and others—who, during the Islamic golden age, served as invaluable conduits of textual transmission and interpretation of Hellenistic learning for an amnesic Europe. First through Sicily and Spain and then via the Crusades, the rich cultural enlightenment of the Islamic world awakened a benighted Europe from its intellectual slumber, and Avicenna was perhaps the movement's greatest ambassador.

Avicenna's continued importance as a towering figure in Islamic history may be seen in his tomb at Hamadan. Even though it had fallen into disrepair by the early 20th century, Osler noted that "the great Persian has still a large practice, as his tomb is much visited by pilgrims, among whom cures are said to be not uncommon." In the 1950s the tomb was refurbished and transformed into an impressive mausoleum adorned with an imposing Mughal-inspired tower, and a museum and 8,000-volume library were added as well. Avicenna's resting place remains a major stop for tourists in the region. Now, as when he was alive, the great physician and philosopher continues to attract the attention of scholars and the public alike.

MOSES MAIMONIDES
(born March 30, 1135, Córdoba [Spain]–died Dec. 13, 1204, Egypt)

Moses Maimonides (original name Moses Ben Maimon), was a Jewish philosopher, jurist, and physician and the foremost intellectual figure of medieval Judaism. His first major work, begun at age 23 and completed 10 years later, was a commentary on the Mishna, the collected Jewish oral laws. A monumental code of Jewish law followed in Hebrew, *The Guide for the Perplexed* in Arabic, and numerous other works, many of major importance. His contributions in religion, philosophy, and medicine have influenced Jewish and non-Jewish scholars alike.

LIFE

Maimonides was born into a distinguished family in Córdoba (Cordova), Spain. The young Moses studied with his learned father, Maimon, and other masters and at an early age astonished his teachers by his remarkable depth and versatility. Before Moses reached his 13th birthday, his peaceful world was suddenly disturbed by the ravages of war and persecution.

As part of Islamic Spain, Córdoba had accorded its citizens full religious freedom. But now the Islamic Mediterranean world was shaken by a revolutionary and fanatical Islamic sect, the Almohads (Arabic: *al-Muwaḥḥidūn*, "the Unitarians"), who captured Córdoba in 1148, leaving the Jewish community faced with the grim alternative of submitting to Islam or leaving the city. The Maimons temporized by practicing their Judaism in the privacy of their homes, while disguising their ways in public as far as possible to appear like Muslims. They remained in Córdoba for some 11 years, and Maimonides continued his education in Judaic studies as well as in the scientific disciplines in vogue at the time.

When the double life proved too irksome to maintain in Córdoba, the Maimon family finally left the city about 1159 to settle in Fez, Morocco. Although it was also under Almohad rule, Fez was presumably more promising than Córdoba because there the Maimons would be strangers, and their disguise would be more likely to go undetected. Moses continued his studies in his favourite subjects, rabbinics and Greek philosophy, and added medicine to them. Fez proved to be no more than a short respite, however. In 1165 Rabbi Judah ibn Shoshan, with whom Moses had studied, was arrested as a practicing Jew and was found guilty and then executed. This was a sign to the Maimon family to move again, this time to Palestine, which was in a depressed economic state and could not offer them the basis of a livelihood. After a few months they moved again, now to Egypt, settling in Fostat, near Cairo. There Jews were free to practice their faith openly, though any Jew who had once submitted to Islam courted death if he relapsed to Judaism. Moses himself was once accused of being a renegade Muslim, but he was able to prove that he had never really adopted the faith of Islam and so was exonerated.

Though Egypt was a haven from harassment and persecution, Moses was soon assailed by personal problems. His father died shortly after the family's arrival in Egypt. His younger brother, David, a prosperous jewelry merchant on whom Moses leaned for support, died in a shipwreck, taking the entire family fortune with him, and Moses was left as the sole support of his family. He could not turn to the rabbinate because in those days the rabbinate was conceived of as a public service that did not offer its practitioners any remuneration. Pressed by economic necessity, Moses took advantage of his medical studies and became a practicing physician. His fame as a physician spread rapidly, and he soon became the court physician to the sultan Saladin, the famous Muslim military leader, and to his son al-Afḍal. He also continued a private practice and lectured before his fellow physicians at the state hospital. At the same time he became the leading member of the Jewish community, teaching in public and helping his people with various personal and communal problems.

Maimonides married late in life and was the father of a son, Abraham, who was to make his mark in his own right in the world of Jewish scholarship.

Works

The writings of Maimonides were numerous and varied. His earliest work, composed in Arabic at the age of 16, was the *Millot ha-Higgayon* ("Treatise on Logical Terminology"), a study of various technical terms that were employed in logic and metaphysics. Another of his early works, also in Arabic, was the "Essay on the Calendar" (Hebrew title: *Ma'amar ha'ibur*).

The first of Maimonides's major works, begun at the age of 23, was his commentary on the Mishna, *Kitāb al-Sirāj*, also written in Arabic. The Mishna is a compendium of decisions in Jewish law that dates from earliest times to the 3rd century. Maimonides's commentary clarified individual words and phrases, frequently citing relevant information in archaeology, theology, or science. Possibly the work's most striking feature is a series of introductory essays dealing with general philosophic issues touched on in the Mishna. One of these essays summarizes the teachings of Judaism in a creed of Thirteen Articles of Faith.

He completed the commentary on the Mishna at the age of 33, after which he began his magnum opus, the code of Jewish law, on which he also laboured for 10 years. Bearing the name of *Mishne Torah* ("The Torah Reviewed") and written in a lucid Hebrew style, the code offers a brilliant systematization of all Jewish law and doctrine. He wrote two other works in Jewish law of lesser scope: the *Sefer ha-mitzwot* (*Book of Precepts*), a digest of law for the less sophisticated reader, written in Arabic; and the "Hilkhot ha-Yerushalmi "("Laws of Jerusalem"), a digest of the laws in the Palestinian Talmud, written in Hebrew.

His next major work, which he began in 1176 and on which he laboured for 15 years, was his classic in religious philosophy, the *Dalālat al-ḥā'irīn* (*The Guide for the Perplexed*), later known under its Hebrew title as the *Moreh nevukhim*. A plea for what he called a more rational philosophy of Judaism, it constituted a major contribution to the accommodation between science, philosophy, and religion. It was written in Arabic and sent as a private communication to his favourite disciple, Joseph ibn Aknin. The work was translated into Hebrew in Maimonides's lifetime and later into Latin and most European languages. It has exerted a marked influence on the history of religious thought.

Maimonides also wrote a number of minor works, occasional essays dealing with current problems that faced the Jewish community, and he maintained an extensive correspondence with scholars, students, and community leaders. Among his minor works those considered to be most important are *Iggert Teman* (*Epistle to Yemen*), *Iggeret ha-shemad* or "Ma'amar Qiddush ha-Shem "("Letter on Apostasy"), and "Iggeret le-qahal Marsilia "("Letter on Astrology," or, literally, "Letter to the Community of Marseille"). He also wrote a number of works dealing with medicine, including a popular miscellany of health rules, which he dedicated to the sultan, al-Afḍal. A mid-20th-century historian, Waldemar Schweisheimer, has said of Maimonides's medical writings: "Maimonides' medical teachings are not antiquated at all. His writings, in fact, are in some respects astonishingly modern in tone and contents."

Maimonides complained often that the pressures of his many duties robbed him of peace and undermined his health. He died in 1204 and was buried in Tiberias, in the Holy Land, where his grave continues to be a shrine drawing a constant stream of pious pilgrims.

Significance

Maimonides's advanced views aroused opposition during his lifetime and after his death. In 1233 one zealot, Rabbi Solomon of Montpellier, in southern France, instigated the church authorities to burn *The Guide for the Perplexed* as a dangerously heretical book. But the controversy abated after some time, and Maimonides came to be recognized as a pillar of the traditional faith—his creed became part of the orthodox liturgy—as well as the greatest of the Jewish philosophers.

Maimonides's epoch-making influence on Judaism extended also to the larger world. His philosophic work, translated into Latin, influenced the great medieval Scholastic writers, and even later thinkers, such as Benedict de Spinoza and G.W. Leibniz, found in his work a source for some of their ideas. His medical writings constitute a significant chapter in the history of medical science.

PARACELSUS

(born Nov. 11 or Dec. 17, 1493, Einsiedeln, Switzerland–died Sept. 24, 1541, Salzburg, Archbishopric of Salzburg [now in Austria])

Paracelsus was the byname of Philippus Aureolus Theophrastus Bombastus Von Hohenheim, a German-Swiss physician and alchemist who established the role of chemistry in medicine. He published *Der grossen Wundartzney* (*Great Surgery Book*) in 1536 and a clinical description of syphilis in 1530.

Education

Paracelsus, who was known as Theophrastus when he was a boy, was the only son of an impoverished German doctor and chemist. His mother died when he was very young, and shortly thereafter his father moved to Villach in southern Austria. There Paracelsus attended the Bergschule, founded by the wealthy Fugger family of merchant bankers of Augsburg, where his father taught chemical theory and practice. Youngsters were trained at the Bergschule as overseers and analysts for mining operations in gold, tin, and mercury, as well as in iron, alum, and copper-sulfate ores.

The young Paracelsus learned of metals that "grow" in the earth, watched the transformations of metallic constituents in smelting vats, and perhaps wondered about the transmutation of lead into gold—a conversion believed to be possible by the alchemists of the time. Those experiences gave Paracelsus insight into metallurgy and chemistry, which likely laid the foundations of his later remarkable discoveries in the field of chemotherapy.

In 1507 Paracelsus joined the many wandering youths who traveled throughout Europe in the late Middle Ages, seeking famous teachers at one university after another.

Paracelsus is said to have attended the Universities of Basel, Tübingen, Vienna, Wittenberg, Leipzig, Heidelberg, and Cologne during the next five years but was disappointed with them all. He wrote later that he wondered how "the high colleges managed to produce so many high asses," a typical Paracelsian jibe.

REJECTION OF TRADITIONAL EDUCATION AND MEDICINE

Paracelsus upset the traditional attitudes of schoolmen. "The universities do not teach all things," he wrote, "so a doctor must seek out old wives, gipsies, sorcerers, wandering tribes, old robbers, and such outlaws and take lessons from them. A doctor must be a traveller....Knowledge is experience." Paracelsus held that the crude language of the innkeeper, the barber, and the teamster had more real dignity and common sense than the dry scholasticism of Aristotle, Galen of Pergamum, and Avicenna, the recognized Greek and Arab medical authorities of his day.

Paracelsus is said to have graduated from the University of Vienna with a baccalaureate in medicine in 1510. He then went to the University of Ferrara in Italy, where he was free to express his rejection of the prevailing view that the stars and the planets controlled all the parts of the human body. It is believed that he received a doctoral degree from the University of Ferrara in 1516, and he is presumed to have begun using the name "para-Celsus" (above or beyond Celsus) at about this time as well. His new name reflected the fact that he regarded himself as even greater than Aulus Cornelius Celsus, a renowned 1st-century Roman medical writer.

Soon after taking his degree, he set out upon many years of wandering through almost every country in Europe, including England, Ireland, and Scotland. He took part in the "Netherlandish wars" as an army surgeon. Later he went to Russia, was held captive by the Tatars, escaped into Lithuania, and went south into Hungary. In 1521 he again served as an army surgeon in Italy. His wanderings eventually took him to Egypt, Arabia, the Holy Land, and, finally, Constantinople. Everywhere he went, he sought out the most learned exponents of practical alchemy, not only to discover the most effective means of medical treatment but also—and even more important—to discover "the latent forces of Nature," and how to use them. He wrote:

> He who is born in imagination discovers the latent forces of Nature.... Besides the stars that are established, there is yet another—*Imagination*—that begets a new star and a new heaven.

Career at Basel

In 1524 Paracelsus returned to his home in Villach to find that his fame for many miraculous cures had preceded him. He was subsequently appointed town physician and lecturer in medicine at the University of Basel in Switzerland, and students from all parts of Europe went to the city to hear his lectures. Pinning a program of his forthcoming lectures to the notice board of the university on June 5, 1527, he invited not only students but anyone and everyone. The authorities were incensed by his open invitation. Ten years earlier German theologian and religious reformer Martin Luther had circulated his Theses on Indulgences. Later, Paracelsus wrote:

> Why do you call me a Medical Luther?...I leave it to Luther to defend what he says, and I will be responsible for what I say. That which you wish to

Luther, you wish also to me: you wish us both in the fire.

Three weeks later, on June 24, 1527, Paracelsus reportedly burned the books of Avicenna, the Arab "Prince of Physicians," and those of the Greek physician Galen, in front of the university. This incident is said to have again recalled in many peoples' minds Luther, who on Dec. 10, 1520, at the Elster Gate of Wittenberg, Germany, had burned a papal bull that threatened excommunication. Paracelsus seemingly remained a Catholic to his death; however, it is suspected that his books were placed on the *Index Expurgatorius* (a catalogue of books from which passages of text considered immoral or against the Catholic religion are removed). Similar to Luther, Paracelsus also lectured and wrote in German rather than in Latin.

Paracelsus reached the peak of his career at Basel. In his lectures, he stressed the healing power of nature and denounced the use of methods of treating wounds, such as padding with moss or dried dung, that prevented natural draining. The wounds must drain, he insisted, for "if you prevent infection, Nature will heal the wound all by herself." He also attacked many other medical malpractices of his time, including the use of worthless pills, salves, infusions, balsams, electuaries, fumigants, and drenches.

However, by the spring of 1528 Paracelsus had fallen into disrepute with local doctors, apothecaries, and magistrates. He left Basel, heading first toward Colmar in Upper Alsace, about 50 miles north of the university. He stayed at various places with friends and continued to travel for the next eight years. During this time, he revised old manuscripts and wrote new treatises. With the publication of *Der grossen Wundartzney* (*Great Surgery*

Book) in 1536 he restored, and even extended, the revered reputation he had earned at Basel. He became wealthy and was sought by royalty.

In May 1538, at the zenith of that second period of renown, Paracelsus returned to Villach again to see his father, only to find that his father had died four years earlier. In 1541 Paracelsus himself died in mysterious circumstances at the White Horse Inn, Salzburg, where he had taken up an appointment under the prince-archbishop, Duke Ernst of Bavaria.

Contributions to Medicine

In 1530 Paracelsus wrote a clinical description of syphilis, in which he maintained that the disease could be successfully treated by carefully measured doses of mercury compounds taken internally. He stated that the "miners' disease" (silicosis) resulted from inhaling metal vapours and was not a punishment for sin administered by mountain spirits. He was the first to declare that, if given in small doses, "what makes a man ill also cures him"—an anticipation of the modern practice of homeopathy. Paracelsus is said to have cured many persons in the plague-stricken town of Stertzing in the summer of 1534 by administering orally a pill made of bread containing a minute amount of the patient's excreta he had removed on a needle point.

Paracelsus was the first to connect goitre with minerals, especially lead, in drinking water. He prepared and used new chemical remedies, including those containing mercury, sulfur, iron, and copper sulfate, thus uniting medicine with chemistry, as the first *London Pharmacopoeia*, in 1618, indicates. Paracelsus, in fact, contributed substantially to the rise of modern medicine, including psychiatric treatment. Swiss psychologist Carl Jung wrote of him that "we see in Paracelsus not only a pioneer in the domains of chemical medicine, but also in those of an empirical psychological healing science."

AMBROISE PARÉ
(born 1510, Bourg-Hersent, France–died Dec. 20, 1590, Paris)

Ambroise Paré was a French physician and one of the most notable surgeons of the European Renaissance, regarded by some medical historians as the father of modern surgery.

About 1533 Paré went to Paris, where he soon became a barber-surgeon apprentice at the Hôtel-Dieu. He was taught anatomy and surgery and in 1537 was employed as an army surgeon. By 1552 he had gained such popularity that he became surgeon to the king; he served four French monarchs: Henry II, Francis II, Charles IX, and Henry III.

At the time Paré entered the army, surgeons treated gunshot wounds with boiling oil since such wounds were believed to be poisonous. On one occasion, when Paré's supply of oil ran out, he treated the wounds with a mixture of egg yolk, rose oil, and turpentine. He found that the wounds he had treated with this mixture were healing better than those treated with the boiling oil. Sometime later he reported his findings in *La Méthod de traicter les playes faites par les arquebuses et aultres bastons à feu* (1545; "The Method of Treating Wounds Made by Harquebuses and Other Guns"), which was ridiculed because it was written in French rather than in Latin. Another of Paré's innovations that did not win immediate medical acceptance was his reintroduction of the tying of large arteries to replace the method of searing vessels with hot irons (i.e., cauterizing) to check hemorrhaging during amputation.

Unlike many surgeons of his time, Paré resorted to surgery only when he found it absolutely necessary. He was one of the first surgeons to discard the practice of castrating patients who required surgery for a hernia. He was the first to describe the sensation of phantom limb syndrome after operating on wounded soldiers who complained of pain in amputated limbs.

Paré introduced the implantation of teeth, artificial limbs, and artificial eyes made of gold and silver. The origin of prosthetics as a science is thus attributed to him. Paré invented many scientific instruments, popularized the use of the truss for hernia, and was the first to suggest syphilis as a cause of aneurysm (swelling of blood vessels). His favourite expression, "I dressed him; God healed him," is characteristic of this humane and careful doctor.

ANDREAS VESALIUS

(born Dec. 1514, Brussels [now in Belgium]–died June 1564, island of Zacynthus, Republic of Venice [now in Greece])

Andreas Vesalius (Flemish Andries Van Wesel) was a Renaissance physician who revolutionized the study of biology and the practice of medicine by his careful description of the anatomy of the human body. Basing his observations on dissections he made himself, he wrote and illustrated the first comprehensive textbook of anatomy.

LIFE

Vesalius, a native of the duchy of Brabant (the southern portion of which is now in Belgium), was from a family of physicians and pharmacists. He attended the Catholic

University of Leuven (Louvain) in 1529–33, and from 1533 to 1536 he studied at the medical school of the University of Paris, where he learned to dissect animals. He also had the opportunity to dissect human cadavers, and he devoted much of his time to a study of human bones, at that time easily available in the Paris cemeteries.

In 1536 Vesalius returned to Brabant to spend another year at the Catholic University of Leuven, where the influence of Arab medicine was still dominant. Following the prevailing custom, he prepared, in 1537, a paraphrase of the work of the 10th-century Arab physician, Rhazes, probably in fulfillment of the requirements for the bachelor of medicine degree. He then went to the University of Padua, a progressive university with a strong tradition of anatomical dissection. On receiving the M.D. degree the same year, he was appointed a lecturer in surgery with the responsibility of giving anatomical demonstrations. Since he knew that a thorough knowledge of human anatomy was essential to surgery, he devoted much of his time to dissections of cadavers and insisted on doing them himself, instead of relying on untrained assistants.

At first, Vesalius had no reason to question the theories of Galen, the Greek physician who had served the emperor Marcus Aurelius in Rome and whose books on anatomy were still considered as authoritative in medical education in Vesalius's time. In January 1540, breaking with this tradition of relying on Galen, Vesalius openly demonstrated his own method—doing dissections himself, learning anatomy from cadavers, and critically evaluating ancient texts. He did so while visiting the University of Bologna. Such methods convinced him that Galenic anatomy had not been based on the dissection of the human body, which had been strictly forbidden by the Roman religion. Galenic anatomy, he maintained, was an application to the human form of conclusions drawn from the dissections of animals, mostly dogs, monkeys, or pigs. It was this conclusion that he had the audacity to declare in his teaching as he hurriedly prepared his complete textbook of human anatomy for publication. Early in 1542 he traveled to Venice to supervise the preparation of drawings to illustrate his text, probably in the studio of the great Renaissance artist Titian. The drawings of his dissections were engraved on wood blocks, which he took, together with his manuscript, to Basel, Switzerland, where his major work *De humani corporis fabrica libri septem* ("The Seven Books on the Structure of the Human Body") commonly known as the *Fabrica*, was printed in 1543.

In this epochal work, Vesalius deployed all his scientific, humanistic, and aesthetic gifts. The *Fabrica* was a more extensive and accurate description of the human body than any put forward by his predecessors; it gave anatomy a new language, and, in the

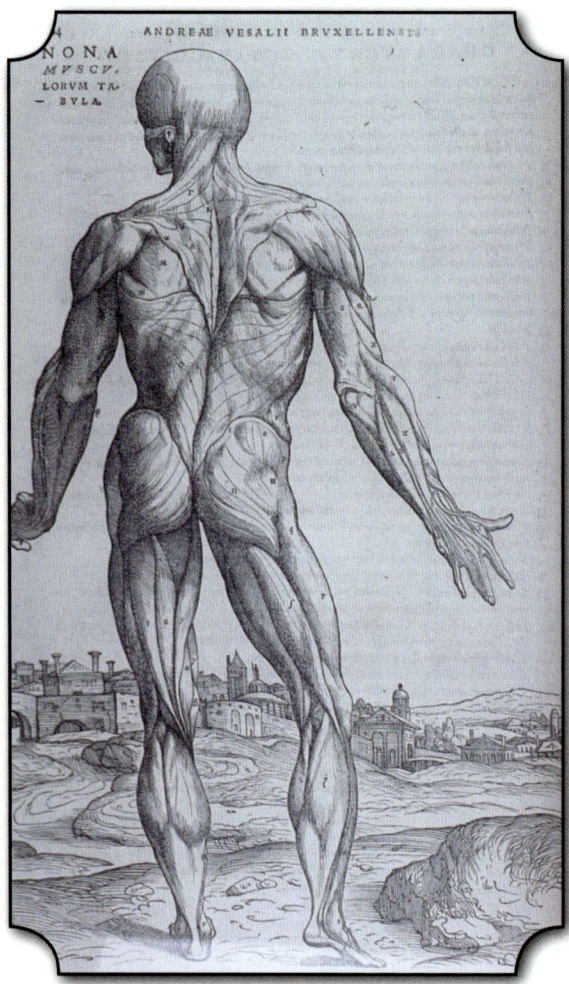

This woodcut illustration of muscles is attributed to the workshop of the Italian painter Titian.

elegance of its printing and organization, a perfection hitherto unknown. Vesalius provided a critical examination of Galen's anatomy and drew on his own studies to correct many of Galen's errors. Like Newton a century later, he emphasized the phenomena—i.e., the accurate description of natural facts.

Early in 1543, Vesalius left for Mainz, to present his book to the Holy Roman emperor Charles V, who engaged him as regular physician to the household. Thus, when not yet 28 years old, Vesalius had attained his goal. After relinquishing his post in Padua, and returning in the spring of 1544 to his native land to marry Anne van Hamme, he took up new duties in the service of the Emperor on his travels in Europe. From 1553 to 1556 Vesalius spent most of his time in Brussels, where he built an imposing house in keeping with his growing affluence and attended to his flourishing medical practice. His prestige was further enhanced when Charles V, on abdication from the Spanish throne in 1556, provided him with a lifetime pension and made him a count.

Vesalius went to Spain in 1559 with his wife and daughter to take up an appointment, made by Philip II, son of Charles V, as one of the physicians in the Madrid court. In 1564 Vesalius obtained permission to leave Spain to go on pilgrimage to the Holy Sepulchre. He traveled to Jerusalem, with stops at Venice and Cyprus, his wife and daughter having returned to Brussels.

Assessment

Vesalius's work represented the culmination of the humanistic revival of ancient learning, the introduction of human dissections into medical curricula, and the growth of a European anatomical literature. Vesalius performed his dissections with a thoroughness hitherto unknown.

Perhaps Vesalius's greatest contribution, however, was that he inspired a group of younger scientists to be critical and to accept a description only after they had verified it.

After Vesalius, anatomy became a scientific discipline, with far-reaching implications not only for physiology but for all of biology. During his own lifetime, however, Vesalius found it easier to correct points of Galenic anatomy than to challenge his physiological framework. Conflicting reports obscure the final days of Vesalius' life. Apparently he became ill aboard ship while returning to Europe from his pilgrimage. He was put ashore on the Greek island of Zacynthus, where he died.

GABRIEL FALLOPIUS
(born 1523, Modena [Italy]–died Oct. 9, 1562, Padua)

Gabriel Fallopius (Italian Gabriello Fallopio *or* Gabriello Fallopia) was the most illustrious of 16th-century Italian anatomists. He contributed greatly to early knowledge of the ear and of the reproductive organs.

Fallopius served as canon of the cathedral of Modena and then turned to the study of medicine at the University of Ferrara, where he became a teacher of anatomy. He then held positions at the University of Pisa (1548–51) and at Padua (1551–62). His exhaustive observations, made during dissection of human cadavers and outlined in *Observationes anatomicae* (1561), earned him the respect and admiration of his colleagues, including the great Renaissance anatomist Andreas Vesalius.

Fallopius discovered the tubes that connect the ovaries to the uterus (now known as fallopian tubes) and several major nerves of the head and face. He described the semicircular canals of the inner ear (responsible for maintaining body equilibrium) and named the vagina, placenta, clitoris, palate, and cochlea (the snail-shaped organ of hearing in the inner ear). A friend and supporter of Vesalius, he joined him in a vigorous assault on the principles of the classic Greek anatomist Galen, which resulted in a shift of attitude essential to the development of Renaissance medicine.

WILLIAM HARVEY

(born April 1, 1578, Folkestone, Kent, England–died June 3, 1657, London)

William Harvey was an English physician who was the first to recognize the full circulation of the blood in the human body and to provide experiments and arguments to support this idea. Before his discoveries blood was thought to ebb and flow through the body by the contraction of arteries. Harvey's work also laid down the foundations of physiology, the study of body functions.

Education and Appointment as Lumleian Lecturer

Harvey had seven brothers and two sisters, and his father, Thomas Harvey, was a farmer and landowner. Harvey attended the King's School in Canterbury, Kent, from 1588 to 1593 and went on to study arts and medicine at Gonville and Caius College, Cambridge, from 1593 to 1599. He continued his studies at the University of Padua, the leading European medical school at the time. He became a student of Italian anatomist and surgeon Hieronymous Fabricius, who had a considerable influence on Harvey. It is also likely that Harvey was taught by Italian philosopher Cesare Cremonini, a prominent follower of Aristotle.

Harvey earned his doctorate from Padua on April 25, 1602, and then returned to England to work as a doctor. In

1604 he married Elizabeth Browne, the daughter of Launcelot Browne, a London physician, who served as physician to James I, the king of England and Scotland. Harvey and his wife appear to have been happy together, and Harvey referred to her as "my dear deceased loving wife" in his will. They did not have any children. Harvey was a fellow of the Royal College of Physicians of London from 1607 and was active in this society for the remainder of his life. In 1615 he was appointed Lumleian lecturer in surgery at the Royal College, a post he held until 1656 (the Lumleian lecture series was named after Lord John Lumley). In 1609 he was appointed physician at St. Bartholomew's Hospital, a post he held until 1643, when the parliamentary authorities in London had him replaced, Harvey being a staunch supporter of the monarchy.

Physician to the King

Harvey was appointed physician to James I in 1618 and continued as physician to Charles I upon Charles's accession to the throne in 1625. Harvey built a considerable practice in this period, tending to many important men, including author and philosopher Sir Francis Bacon. In 1625 Harvey led the group of doctors attending James during his last illness and was an important witness in the trial of George Villiers, duke of Buckingham, who was accused of poisoning the king. Harvey was rewarded by Charles I for his care of James. Charles and Harvey seem to have enjoyed an amicable relationship, Harvey being allowed to experiment on the royal herd of deer and presenting interesting medical cases to the king.

Harvey lived during the European witch hunt. He was involved in one of the cases, in 1634, and had to examine four women accused of witchcraft. At a time when belief in witches was commonplace and to deny their existence was heresy, it would have been very easy to interpret any suspicious behaviour or mark on the body as positive evidence of witchcraft. It is much to Harvey's credit that he treated the case with an open mind and was willing to consider scientific explanations of the evidence allegedly showing witchcraft. The alleged witches were found to be innocent.

In 1636 Harvey acted as doctor to a diplomatic mission sent to see the Holy Roman emperor, Ferdinand II. This involved nearly a year of travel around Europe. He met renowned German professor of medicine Casper Hofmann at Nürnberg and attempted to demonstrate the circulation of the blood to him. Harvey also had a wide interest in philosophy, literature, and art. During the diplomatic mission of 1636 he visited Italy to look for paintings for the royal collection. He was friends with Robert Fludd, an important English physician and philosopher whose primary interest concerned natural magic, and Thomas Hobbes, a famous political philosopher. He was also acquainted with John Aubrey, the 17th-century biographer, who gave an account of Harvey in his manuscript *Brief Lives*.

Harvey was a committed royalist. He followed the king on the Scottish campaigns of 1639, 1640, and 1641, was with him from 1642 to 1646 during the English Civil Wars, and was even present at the Battle of Edgehill in 1642. His political views may be judged from the dedication to the king in his most important book, *De Motu Cordis* (1628):

> Most serene King! The animal's heart is the basis of its life, its chief member, the sun of its microcosm; on the heart all its activity depends, from the heart all its liveliness and strength arise. Equally is the king the basis of his kingdoms, the sun of his

microcosm, the heart of the state; from him all power arises and all grace stems.

Harvey attended Charles in Oxford during the Civil Wars and in Newcastle when the king was held in captivity. Harvey eventually returned to London, in 1647.

LATER LIFE

In Harvey's later life, he suffered from gout, kidney stones, and insomnia. In 1651, following the publication of his final work, *Exercitationes de Generatione Animalium* (*Exercises on the Generation of Animals*), it is believed that Harvey attempted to take his own life with laudanum (an alcoholic tincture of opium). However, this attempt failed. On June 3, 1657, at the age of 79, he died of a stroke.

One of the worst setbacks Harvey experienced concerned the loss of a great deal of written work when parliamentary troops ransacked his house in Whitehall in 1642. He considered the loss of his book on the generation of insects, which contained the results of a great amount of research, to be the "greatest crucifying" that he had in his life. He also lost notes on patients, postmortem examinations, and animal dissections. Further material was lost in the Great Fire of London in 1666, which engulfed the library that Harvey helped establish at the Royal College of Physicians.

DISCOVERY OF CIRCULATION

Harvey's key work was *Exercitatio Anatomica de Motu Cordis et Sanguinis in Animalibus* (*Anatomical Exercise on the Motion of the Heart and Blood in Animals*), published in

1628, with an English version in 1653. Harvey's greatest achievement was to recognize that the blood flows rapidly around the human body, being pumped through a single system of arteries and veins, and to support this hypothesis with experiments and arguments. There had been suggestions, both within the European tradition (by 16th-century Spanish physician Servetus) and within the Islamic tradition (by 13th-century Muslim physician Ibn an-Nafīs) of a "lesser circulation," whereby blood circulated from the heart to the lungs and back, without circulating around the whole body.

Prior to Harvey, it was believed there were two separate blood systems in the body. One carried purple, "nutritive" blood and used the veins to distribute nutrition from the liver to the rest of the body. The other carried scarlet, "vivyfying" (or "vital") blood and used the arteries to distribute a life-giving principle from the lungs. Today these blood systems are understood as deoxygenated blood and oxygenated blood. However, at the time, the influence of oxygen on blood was not understood. Furthermore, blood was not thought to circulate around the body—it was believed to be consumed by the body at the same rate that it was produced. The capillaries, small vessels linking the arteries and veins, were unknown at the time, and their existence was not confirmed until later in the 17th century, after Harvey, when the microscope had been invented.

Harvey claimed he was led to his discovery of the circulation by consideration of the venous valves. It was known that there were small flaps inside the veins that allowed free passage of blood in one direction but strongly inhibited the flow of blood in the opposite direction. It was thought that these flaps prevented pooling of the blood under the influence of gravity, but

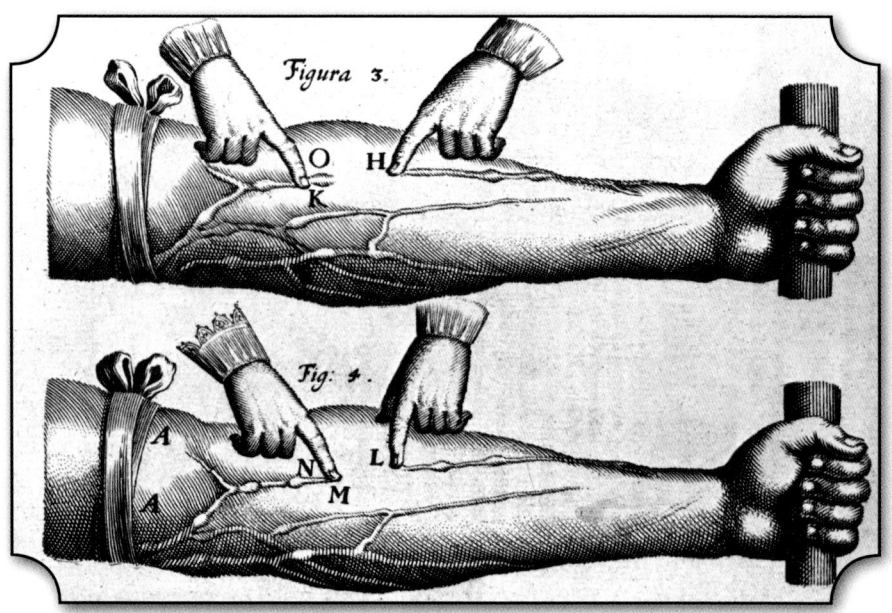

This woodcut depicts William Harvey's theory of the circulation of blood.

Harvey was able to show that all these flaps are cardiocentrically oriented. For example, he showed that in the jugular vein of the neck they face downward, inhibiting blood flow away from the heart, instead of upward, inhibiting pooling due to gravity.

Harvey's main experiment concerned the amount of blood flowing through the heart. He made estimates of the volume of the ventricles, how efficient they were in expelling blood, and the number of beats per minute made by the heart. He was able to show, even with conservative estimates, that more blood passed through the heart than could possibly be accounted for based on the then current understanding of blood flow. Harvey's values indicated the heart pumped 0.5–1 litre of blood per minute (modern values are about 4 litres per minute at rest and 25 litres per minute during exercise). The human body contains about 5 litres of blood. The body simply could not produce or consume that amount of blood so rapidly; therefore, the blood had to circulate.

It is also important that Harvey investigated the nature of the heartbeat. Prior to Harvey, it was thought that the active phase of the heartbeat, when the muscles contract, was when the heart increased its internal volume. So the active motion of the heart was to draw blood into itself. Harvey observed the heart beating in many animals—particularly in cold-blooded animals and in animals near death, because their heartbeats were slow. He concluded that the active phase of the heartbeat, when the muscles contract, is when the heart decreases its internal volume and that blood is expelled with considerable force from the heart.

It is tempting to view Harvey, with his quantitative experiment and his model of the heart as a pump, as someone who supported or was inspired by the new mathematical and mechanical ideas of the 17th century, which played significant roles in the scientific revolution of the time. However, there is a need for considerable caution here. Harvey did quantify blood flow, but his quantification is very approximate, and he deliberately used underestimates to further his case. This is very different from the precise quantification leading to the mathematical laws of someone like Galileo. It was important that Harvey saw the heart as a pump, but he saw it as an organic pump, rather than as a mechanical pump. He also interpreted the blood as having an irreducible life force of its own. Harvey was deeply and bitterly opposed to the mechanical philosophy of French mathematician and philosopher René Descartes as well as to any purely mechanical conception of the human body.

Harvey's theory of circulation was opposed by conservative physicians, but it was well established by the time of his death. It is likely that Harvey actually made his discovery of the circulation about 1618–19. Such a major shift in thinking about the body needed to be very well supported by experiment and argument to avoid immediate ridicule and dismissal; hence the delay before the publication of his central work. In 1649 Harvey published *Exercitationes Duae Anatomicae de Circulatione Sanguinis, ad Joannem Riolanem, Filium, Parisiensem* (*Two Anatomical Exercises on the Circulation of the Blood*) in response to criticism of the circulation theory by French anatomist Jean Riolan.

Renaissance Influences

Harvey was very much influenced by the ideas of Greek philosopher Aristotle and the natural magic tradition of the Renaissance. His key analogy for the circulation of the blood was a macrocosm/microcosm analogy with the weather system. A macrocosm/microcosm analogy sees similarities between a small system and a large system. Thus, one might say that the solar system is a macrocosm and the atom is a microcosm. The Renaissance natural magic tradition was very keen on the idea of the human body as a microcosm. The macrocosm for Harvey was the Earth's weather cycle. Water was changed into vapour by the action of the Sun, and the vapour rose, was cooled, and fell again as rain. The microcosm was the human body, where the action of the heart was supposed to heat and change the blood, which was cooled again in the extremities of the body. Harvey says (and compare the earlier quote concerning the king) that:

So the heart is the beginning of life, the Sun of the Microcosm, as proportionably the Sun deserves to be call'd the heart of the world, by whose vertue, and pulsation, the blood is mov'd, perfected, made vegetable, and is defended from corruption and mattering; and this familiar household-god doth his duty to the whole body, by nourishing, cherishing, and vegetating, being the foundation of life, and author of all.

This was critical to Harvey. How could arterial blood be rapidly, efficiently, and consistently converted into venous blood (and vice versa) within one system? This was a key question, which prompted Harvey to draw on his macrocosm/microcosm analogy. It also should be noted that much of his terminology for change was drawn from the alchemy of his time. Harvey was very much a man of the later Renaissance—not a man of the scientific revolution and its mechanical nature.

Studies of Reproduction

Harvey spent much of the latter part of his career working on the nature of reproduction in animals. He worked on chickens as an example of oviparous reproduction, in which embryonic development occurs within eggs hatched outside the mother's body, and on deer as an example of viviparous reproduction, in which embryonic development occurs within the mother's body, resulting in the birth of live young. Harvey's work in this area generated a wealth of observational detail. At the time, reproduction was poorly understood, and Harvey investigated issues of the role of sperm and menstrual blood in the formation of the embryo. His observations were excellent, but such matters could not be resolved properly without the use of the microscope.

THOMAS SYDENHAM
(born 1624, Wynford Eagle, Dorset, England–died Dec. 29, 1689, London)

Thomas Sydenham was a physician who is recognized as a founder of clinical medicine and epidemiology. Because he emphasized detailed observations of patients and maintained accurate records, he has been called "the English Hippocrates."

Although his medical studies at the University of Oxford were interrupted by his participation on the parliamentary side during the first of the English Civil Wars, Sydenham received his M.B. in 1648 and began to practice about 1656 in London, where he made an exacting study of epidemics. This work formed the basis of his book on fevers (1666), later expanded into *Observationes Medicae* (1676), a standard textbook for two centuries. His treatise on gout (1683) is considered his masterpiece.

He was among the first to describe scarlet fever—differentiating it from measles and naming it—and to explain the nature of hysteria and St. Vitus's Dance (Sydenham chorea). Sydenham chorea is a neurological disorder characterized by irregular and involuntary movements of muscle groups in various parts of the body that follow streptococcal infection. The name St. Vitus's Dance derives from the late Middle Ages, when persons with the disease attended the chapels of St. Vitus, who was believed to have curative powers. Most often a manifestation of rheumatic fever, Sydenham chorea occurs most frequently between the ages of 5 and 15 years, and is more common in girls than boys. The disease may occur as an infrequent complication of pregnancy.

The symptoms of Sydenham chorea range in severity from mild to completely incapacitating. A vague deterioration in the ability to perform everyday tasks is replaced by involuntary jerking movements that are most obvious in the extremities and face but are also present in the trunk. Twitching movements are more noticeable on the limbs of one side of the body. The muscles of speech and swallowing may also be affected. Irritability, anxiety, and emotional instability, chiefly episodes of crying initiated by trivial incidents, are also common symptoms.

It is thought that Sydenham chorea is caused by a malfunctioning of the basal ganglia, groups of nerve cells in the brain. There is evidence that both the emotional manifestations and the abnormal movements of the disease are related to changes in the cerebral cortex. Attacks of Sydenham chorea tend to be self-limited, although the duration of each is several weeks; recurrence is frequent. Recovery is usually complete and is accelerated by bedrest. Sedation or the administration of tranquilizers may provide protection from self-injury in severe cases, when the patient is helpless.

Sydenham introduced laudanum (alcohol tincture of opium) into medical practice, was one of the first to use iron in treating iron-deficiency anemia, and helped popularize quinine in treating malaria.

Derided by his colleagues, Sydenham benefited immensely from a consequent detachment from the speculative theories of his time. Sydenham was not a voluminous writer and, indeed, had little patience with book learning in medicine; nevertheless, he gave excellent descriptions of the phenomena of disease. His greatest service, much needed at the time, was to divert physicians' minds from speculation and lead them back to the bedside, where the true art of medicine could be studied.

MARCELLO MALPIGHI
(born March 10, 1628, Crevalcore, near Bologna, Papal States [Italy]–died Nov. 30, 1694, Rome)

Marcello Malpighi was an Italian physician and biologist who, in developing experimental methods to study living things, founded the science of microscopic anatomy. After Malpighi's researches, microscopic anatomy became a prerequisite for advances in the fields of physiology, embryology, and practical medicine.

LIFE

Little is known of Malpighi's childhood and youth except that his father had him engage in "grammatical studies" at an early age and that he entered the University of Bologna in 1646. Both parents died when he was 21, but he was able, nevertheless, to continue his studies. Despite opposition from the university authorities because he was non-Bolognese by birth, in 1653 he was granted doctorates in both medicine and philosophy and appointed as a teacher, whereupon he immediately dedicated himself to further study in anatomy and medicine.

In 1656, Ferdinand II of Tuscany invited him to the professorship of theoretical medicine at the University of Pisa. There Malpighi began his lifelong friendship with Giovanni Borelli, mathematician and naturalist, who was a prominent supporter of the Accademia del Cimento, one of the first scientific societies. Malpighi questioned the prevailing medical teachings at Pisa, tried experiments on colour changes in blood, and attempted to recast anatomical, physiological, and medical problems of the day. Family responsibilities and poor health prompted Malpighi's return in 1659 to the University of Bologna, where he continued to teach and do research with his microscopes. In 1661 he identified and described the pulmonary and capillary network connecting small arteries with small veins, one of the major discoveries in the history of science. Malpighi's views evoked increasing controversy and dissent, mainly from envy, jealousy, and lack of understanding on the part of his colleagues.

Hindered by the hostile environment of Bologna, Malpighi accepted (November 1662) a professorship in medicine at the University of Messina in Sicily, on the recommendation there of Borelli, who was investigating the effects of physical forces on animal functions. Malpighi was also welcomed by Visconte Giacomo Ruffo Francavilla, a patron of science and a former student, whose hospitality encouraged him in furthering his career. Malpighi pursued his microscopic studies while teaching and practicing medicine. He identified the taste buds and regarded them as terminations of nerves, described the minute structure of the brain, optic nerve, and fat reservoirs, and in 1666 was the first to see the red blood cells and to attribute the colour of blood to them. Again, his research and teaching aroused envy and controversy among his colleagues.

After four years at Messina, Malpighi returned in January 1667 to Bologna, where, during his medical practice, he studied the microscopic subdivisions of specific living organs, such as the liver, brain, spleen, and kidneys, and of bone and the deeper layers of the skin that now bear his name. Impressed by the minute structures he observed under the microscope, he concluded that most living materials are glandular in organization, that even the largest organs are composed of minute glands, and that these glands exist solely for the separation or for the mixture of juices.

Malpighi's work at Messina attracted the attention of the Royal Society in London, whose secretary, Henry Oldenburg, extended him an invitation in 1668 to correspond with him. Malpighi's work was thereafter published periodically in the form of letters in the *Philosophical Transactions* of the Royal Society. In 1669 Malpighi was named an honorary member, the first such recognition given to an Italian. From then on, all his works were published in London.

At the peak of his fame, Malpighi could have left his tiring medical practice and research to accept one of the many highly remunerative positions offered to him. Instead, he chose to continue his general practice and professorship. His years at Bologna marked the climax of his career, when he marked out large areas of microscopy. Malpighi conducted many studies of insect larvae—establishing, in so doing, the basis for their future study—the most important of which was his investigation in 1669 of the structure and development of the silkworm. In his historic work in 1673 on the embryology of the chick, in which he discovered the aortic arches, neural folds, and somites, he generally followed William Harvey's views on development, though Malpighi probably concluded that the embryo is preformed in the egg after fertilization. He also made extensive comparative studies in 1675–79 of the microscopic anatomy of several different plants and saw an analogy between plant and animal organization.

During the last decade of his life Malpighi was beset by personal tragedy, declining health, and the climax of opposition to him. In 1684 his villa was burned, his apparatus and microscopes shattered, and his papers, books, and manuscripts destroyed. Most probably as a compensatory move when opposition mounted against his views, and in recognition of his stature, Pope Innocent XII invited him to Rome in 1691 as papal archiater, or personal physician, such a nomination constituting a great honour. In Rome he was further honoured by being named a count, he was elected to the College of Doctors of Medicine, his name was placed in the Roman Patriciate Roll, and he was given the title of honorary valet.

Assessment

Malpighi may be regarded as the first histologist (histology being the microscopic study of the structure, composition, and function of tissues). For almost 40 years he used the microscope to describe the major types of plant and animal structures and in so doing marked out for future generations of biologists major areas of research in botany, embryology, human anatomy, and pathology. He was the first to describe the inner (malpighian) layer of the skin, the papillae of the tongue, the outer part (cortex) of the cerebral area of the brain, and the red blood cells. He also wrote a detailed monograph on the silkworm. In addition to those, Malpighi made detailed investigations in plant anatomy. He systematically described the various parts of plants, such as bark, stem, roots, and seeds, and discussed processes such as germination and gall formation. Many of Malpighi's drawings of plant anatomy remained unintelligible to botanists until the structures were rediscovered in the 19th century. Just as Galileo had applied the new technical achievement of the optical lens to vistas beyond the Earth, Malpighi extended its use to the intricate organization of living things, hitherto unimagined, below the level of unaided sight.

Moreover, his lifework brought into question the prevailing concepts of body function. When, for example, he found that the blood passed through the capillaries, it meant that Harvey was right, that blood was not transformed into flesh in the periphery, as the ancients thought. He was vigorously denounced by his enemies, who failed to see how his many discoveries, such as the renal glomeruli, urinary tubules, dermal papillae, taste buds, and the glandular components of the liver, could possibly improve medical practice. The conflict between ancient ideas and modern discoveries continued throughout the 17th century. Although Malpighi could not say what new remedies might come from his discoveries, he was convinced that microscopic anatomy, by showing the minute construction of living things, called into question the value of old medicine. He provided the anatomical basis for the eventual understanding of human physiological exchanges.

Although Malpighi was not a technical innovator, he does exemplify the functioning of the educated 17th-century mind, which, together with curiosity and patience, resulted in many advances in biology.

ANTONIE VAN LEEUWENHOEK
(born Oct. 24, 1632, Delft, Netherlands–died Aug. 26, 1723, Delft)

Antonie van Leeuwenhoek was a Dutch microscopist who was the first to observe bacteria and protozoa. His researches on lower animals refuted the doctrine of spontaneous generation, and his observations helped lay the foundations for the sciences of bacteriology and protozoology.

Little is known of Leeuwenhoek's early life. When his stepfather died in 1648, he was sent to Amsterdam to be an apprentice to a linen draper. Returning to Delft when he was 20, he established himself as a draper and haberdasher. In 1660 he obtained a position as chamberlain to the sheriffs of Delft. His income was thus secure and sufficient enough to enable him to devote much of his time to his all-absorbing hobby, that of grinding lenses and using them to study tiny objects.

The magnifying power of segments of glass spheres was known to the Assyrians before the time of Christ; during the 2nd century CE, Claudius Ptolemy, an astronomer, mathematician, and geographer at Alexandria, wrote a treatise on optics in which he discussed the phenomena of magnification and refraction as related to such lenses and to glass spheres filled with water. Despite that knowledge, however, glass lenses were not used extensively until around 1300 (an anonymous person invented spectacles for the improvement of vision probably in the late 1200s). That invention aroused curiosity concerning the property of lenses to magnify, and in the 16th century several papers were written about such devices. Then, in the late 16th century, the Dutch optician Hans Jansen and his son Zacharias invented the compound microscope. The utility of that instrument in the biological sciences, however, was not realized until the following century. Following subsequent technological improvements in the instrument and the development of a more-liberal attitude toward scientific research, five microscopists emerged who were to have a profound affect on biology: Marcello Malpighi, Antonie van Leeuwenhoek, Jan Swammerdam, Nehemiah Grew, and Robert Hooke.

Leeuwenhoek made microscopes consisting of a single, high-quality lens of very short focal length; at the time, such simple microscopes were preferable to the compound microscope, which increased the problem of chromatic aberration. Leeuwenhoek achieved

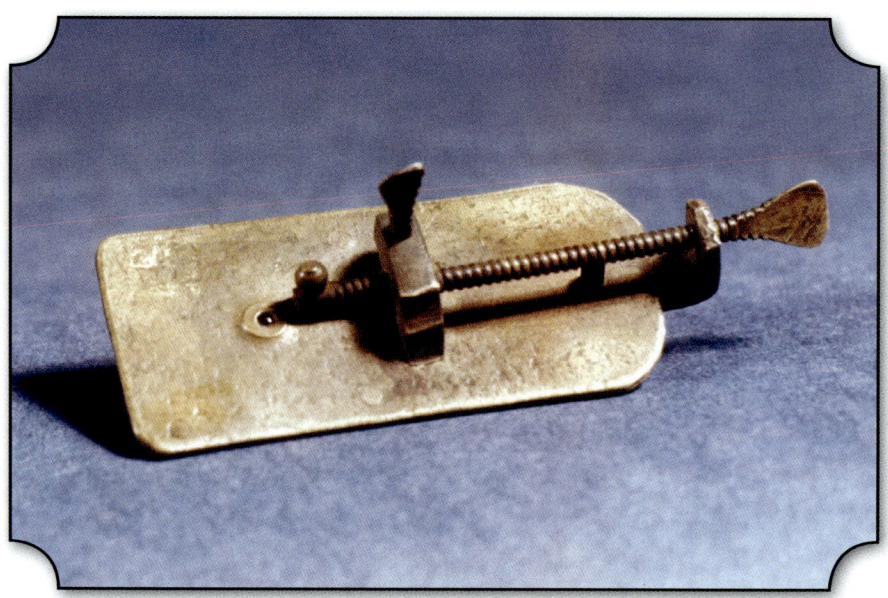

Antonie van Leeuwenhoek's microscope had a small but precise lens that was held up close to the eye in order to view a specimen.

magnifications from 40 to 270 diameters, a remarkable feat for hand-ground lenses. Although Leeuwenhoek's studies lacked the organization of formal scientific research, his powers of careful observation enabled him to make discoveries of fundamental importance. In 1674 he began to observe bacteria and protozoa, his "very little animalcules," which he was able to isolate from different sources, such as rainwater, pond and well water, and the human mouth and intestine, and he calculated their sizes.

In 1677 he described for the first time the spermatozoa from insects, dogs, and man, though Stephen Hamm probably was a codiscoverer. Furthermore, he discovered spermatozoa in the female tract following copulation; the latter destroyed the idea held by others that the entire future development of an animal is centred in the egg, and that sperm merely induce a "vapour," which penetrates the womb and effects fertilization. Although that theory of preformation, as it is called, continued to survive for some time longer, Leeuwenhoek initiated its eventual demise.

Leeuwenhoek studied the structure of the optic lens, striations in muscles, the mouthparts of insects, and the fine structure of plants and discovered parthenogenesis in aphids. In 1680 he noticed that yeasts consist of minute globular particles. He extended Marcello Malpighi's demonstration in 1660 of the blood capillaries by giving (in 1684) the first accurate description of red blood cells. In his observations on rotifers in 1702, Leeuwenhoek remarked that "in all falling rain, carried from gutters into water-butts, animalcules are to be found; and that in all kinds of water, standing in the open air, animalcules can turn up. For these animalcules can be carried over by the wind, along with the bits of dust floating in the air."

A friend of Leeuwenhoek put him in touch with the Royal Society of England, to which, from 1673 until 1723, he communicated by means of informal letters most of his discoveries and to which he was elected a fellow in 1680. His discoveries were for the most part made public in the society's *Philosophical Transactions*. The first representation of bacteria is to be found in a drawing by Leeuwenhoek in that publication in 1683.

His researches on the life histories of various low forms of animal life were in opposition to the doctrine that they could be produced spontaneously or bred from corruption. The theory of spontaneous generation, held by the ancient world and passed down unquestioned, was now being criticized. According to this theory, pieces of cheese and bread wrapped in rags and left in a dark corner, for example, were thus thought to produce mice, because after several weeks there were mice in the rags. Many believed in spontaneous generation because it explained such occurrences as the appearance of maggots on decaying meat. Christiaan Huygens, a scientific friend of Leeuwenhoek, hypothesized that the little animals might be small enough to float in the air and, on reaching water, reproduce themselves. At the time, however, criticism of spontaneous generation went no farther.

Leeuwenhoek showed that the weevils (common pests) that were found in granaries (storehouses for grain) are really grubs hatched from eggs deposited by winged insects. Prior to this, it was commonly supposed that weevils were bred from wheat as well as in it. His letter on the flea, in which he not only described its structure but traced out the whole history of its metamorphosis, is of great interest, not so much for the exactness of his observations as for an illustration of his opposition to the spontaneous generation of many lower organisms, such as "this minute and despised creature." Some theorists asserted that the flea was produced from sand, others from dust or the like, but Leeuwenhoek proved that it bred in the regular way of winged insects.

Leeuwenhoek also carefully studied the history of the ant and was the first to show that what had been commonly reputed to be ants' eggs were really their pupae, containing the perfect insect nearly ready for emergence, and that the true eggs were much smaller and gave origin to maggots, or larvae. He argued that the sea mussel and other shellfish were not generated out of sand found at the seashore or mud in the beds of rivers at low water but from spawn, by the regular course of generation. He maintained the same to be true of the freshwater mussel, whose embryos he examined so carefully that he was able to observe how they were consumed by "animalcules," many of which, according to his description, must have included ciliates in conjugation, flagellates, and the

Vorticella. Similarly, he investigated the generation of eels, which were at that time supposed to be produced from dew without the ordinary process of generation.

The dramatic nature of his discoveries made him world famous, and he was visited by many notables—including Peter I the Great of Russia, James II of England, and Frederick II the Great of Prussia.

Leeuwenhoek's methods of microscopy, which he kept secret, remain something of a mystery. During his lifetime he ground more than 400 lenses, most of which were very small—some no larger than a pinhead—and usually mounted them between two thin brass plates, riveted together. A large sample of these lenses, bequeathed to the Royal Society, were found to have magnifying powers of between 50 and, at the most, 300 times. In order to observe phenomena as small as bacteria, Leeuwenhoek must have employed some form of oblique illumination (lighting from one side), or other technique, for enhancing the effectiveness of the lens, but this method he would not reveal. Leeuwenhoek continued his work almost to the end of his long life of 90 years.

Leeuwenhoek's contributions to the *Philosophical Transactions* amounted to 375 and those to the *Memoirs of the Paris Academy of Sciences* to 27. Two collections of his works appeared during his life, one in Dutch (1685–1718) and the other in Latin (1715–22); a selection was translated by S. Hoole, *The Select Works of A. van Leeuwenhoek* (1798–1807).

WILLIAM CHESELDEN

(born Oct. 19, 1688, Somerby, Leicestershire, England–died April 10, 1752, Bath, Somersetshire)

William Cheselden was a British surgeon and teacher of anatomy and surgery, who wrote *Anatomy of the*

Human Body (1713) and *Osteographia, or the Anatomy of the Bones* (1733). The former was used as a text by anatomy students for nearly a century.

Cheselden was apprenticed to a Mr. Wilkes, surgeon of Leicester. He also studied under the anatomist William Cowper in 1703 and under James Ferne, a surgeon and lithotomist (specialist in removal of bladder stones) at St. Thomas' Hospital. By 1711 he was already established as a lecturer in anatomy. Cheselden was named assistant surgeon at St. Thomas' in 1718 and was elected one of the institution's principal surgeons the following year. Queen Caroline appointed him to be her surgeon in 1727. In 1733 he published *Osteographia,* an atlas of the bones of the human body that was widely celebrated for the beauty and accuracy of its illustrations.

Cheselden was known for his swift and skillful operations; it was reported that he could perform a lithotomy in 54 seconds. He was, in 1727, the first surgeon to extract bladder stones using the lateral (rather than the suprapubic [from above the pubic bone]) approach, a technique invented by him and soon used by surgeons throughout Europe. The following year he surgically restored a blind man's vision and devised a method of treatment for some forms of blindness in which an opening, created by surgery, functioned as an "artificial pupil."

SIR PERCIVALL POTT
(born Jan. 6, 1714, London, England–died Dec. 22, 1788, London)

Percivall Pott was an English surgeon noted for his many insightful and comprehensive surgical writings. He was the first to associate cancer with occupational exposure.

Pott, whose father died when he was a young boy, was raised under the care of his mother and a relative, Joseph Wilcocks, the bishop of Rochester. He was sent to a private school in Kent and later was an apprentice to Edward Nourse, a surgeon at St. Bartholomew's Hospital in London. In preparing and dissecting cadavers for Nourse's anatomy classes, Pott not only became educated in the basic principles of anatomy and medicine but also eventually perfected his surgical technique. In 1736, after seven years under Nourse's instruction, Pott passed examinations for admittance to the Company of Barber Surgeons—the forerunner of the Royal College of Surgeons of England. The Company awarded Pott the Grand Diploma, an honorary achievement, in recognition of his exceptional surgical skills. In 1745 he became an assistant surgeon at St. Bartholomew's and was promoted to full surgeon in 1749.

In 1756, while on his way to see a patient, Pott was thrown from his horse and sustained an open compound fracture of his lower leg. He refused to allow his rescuers to move him right away. Instead, he instructed them to build a makeshift stretcher from a door and poles, which was used to carry him home. Several of his surgical colleagues examined the injury and recommended amputation, the standard course of treatment at the time. Nourse, however, who also went to see Pott, advised otherwise, suggesting reduction, in which traction and pressure are applied to the fracture to correct the positioning of the bones. Nourse's technique worked, and Pott's leg healed without complication. The reduction approach introduced by Nourse was subsequently refined and became widely used in the treatment of open compound fracture, leading to a substantial decline in amputations. In addition, fractures of the lower leg similar to the type Pott suffered became known as Pott fracture. During his recovery, Pott wrote *A Treatise on Ruptures* (1756), a medical work in which he disproved misguided theories on the causes and treatment of hernias.

In *Chirurgical Observations Relative to the Cataract, the Polyplus of the Nose, the Cancer of the Scrotum, the Different Kinds of Ruptures, and the Mortification of the Toes and Feet* (1775), Pott published the first report of cancer caused by occupational exposure. He observed an unusually high incidence of skin sores on the scrotums of men working as chimney sweeps in London. He also discovered coal soot in the sores and eventually concluded that men routinely exposed to soot were at a high risk for scrotal cancer. Pott hypothesized that tumours in the skin of the scrotum were caused by prolonged contact with ropes that were saturated with chemicals found in soot. He noted that some men with scrotal cancer had not worked as chimney sweeps since boyhood—an observation suggesting that cancer develops slowly and may not give rise to clinical manifestations until long after exposure to a causal agent. Pott's report was the first in which an environmental factor was identified as a cancer-causing agent. The disease became known as chimney-sweepers' cancer, and Pott's work laid the foundation for occupational medicine and measures to prevent work-related disease.

Pott also described a disease of the vertebrae in which the bones soften and collapse, causing the spine to curve and produce a hunched back. The condition, Pott disease, is now known to result from infection with the tuberculosis organism *Mycobacterium tuberculosis*. The infection begins in the body of the vertebra (the most common site of bone tuberculosis) and spreads slowly to contiguous structures. Abscesses may form and drain into soft tissues adjacent to the spine, causing pain in sites distant from the infection. Occasionally the spinal nerves are affected, and paralysis may result. Affected persons complain of pain on movement and tend to assume a protective, stiff position. The course of the disease is slow, lasting months or years. Treatment includes chemotherapy against the *M. tuberculosis* bacillus and orthopedic care of the spinal column. Modern treatment has made Pott disease rare in developed countries, but in less-developed countries it still accounts for up to 2 percent of all tuberculosis cases and particularly affects children.

JAMES LIND
(born 1716, Edinburgh, Scotland–died July 13, 1794, Gosport, Hampshire, England)

James Lind was a physician known as the "founder of naval hygiene in England." His recommendation that fresh citrus fruit and lemon juice be included in the diet of seamen eventually resulted in the eradication of scurvy from the British Navy.

A British naval surgeon (1739–48) and a physician at the Haslar Hospital for men of the Royal Navy, Gosport (1758–94), Lind observed thousands of cases of scurvy, typhus, and dysentery and the conditions on board ship that caused them. In 1754, when he published *A Treatise on Scurvy*, more British sailors were dying from scurvy during wartime than were killed in combat.

Scurvy is one of the oldest-known nutritional disorders of humankind. It is caused by a dietary lack of vitamin C (ascorbic acid), a nutrient found in many fresh fruits and vegetables, particularly the citrus fruits. Vitamin C is important in the formation of collagen (an element of normal tissues), and any deficiency of the vitamin interferes with normal tissue synthesis, a problem that underlies the clinical manifestations of the disorder. Scurvy is characterized by swollen and bleeding gums with loosened teeth, soreness and stiffness of the joints and lower extremities, bleeding under the skin and in deep tissues, slow wound healing, and anemia. Although accounts of what was probably scurvy are found in ancient writings, the first clear-cut descriptions appear in the records of the medieval Crusades.

In an early example of a clinical trial, Lind compared the effects of citrus fruits on patients with scurvy against five alternative remedies, showing that the fruit was noticeably better than vinegar, cider, seawater, and other remedies. Selecting 12 sailors who were ill with scurvy, Lind divided them into pairs, each pair receiving a different dietary supplement. One of the pairs was given lemons and oranges to eat, and within a week the two sailors' symptoms had disappeared. The symptoms of the sailors on the other dietary regimens, however, persisted.

Nearly two centuries earlier the Dutch had discovered the benefits of citrus fruits and juices to sailors on long voyages. In his *Treatise* and in *On the Most Effectual Means of Preserving the Health of Seamen* (1757), Lind recommended this dietary practice. His findings ultimately influenced the decision by the British navy to make lemon juice (later replaced by lime juice) a compulsory part of sailors' diets. When it was finally adopted by the Royal Navy in 1795, scurvy disappeared from the ranks "as if by magic." Lind recommended shipboard delousing procedures, suggested the use of hospital ships for sick sailors in tropical ports, and arranged (1761) for the shipboard distillation of seawater for drinking. He also wrote *An Essay on Diseases Incidental to Europeans in Hot Climates* (1768).

JOHN HUNTER

(born Feb. 13, 1728, Long Calderwood, Lanarkshire, Scotland–died Oct. 16, 1793, London, England)

John Hunter was a surgeon who founded pathological anatomy in England. He was an early advocate of investigation and experimentation. He also carried out many important studies and experiments in comparative aspects of biology, anatomy, physiology, and pathology.

Hunter never completed a course of studies in any university, and, as was common for surgeons during the 18th century, he never attempted to become a doctor of medicine. He went to London in 1748 to assist in the preparation of dissections for the course of anatomy taught by his brother William, a famed obstetrician. For 11 winters he studied anatomy in his brother's dissecting rooms, and in the summers of 1749 and 1750 he learned surgery from William Cheselden at Chelsea Hospital.

In 1753 he was elected a master of anatomy at Surgeon's Hall, responsible for reading lectures. He began his own private lectures on the principles and practice of surgery in the early 1770s. In addition, he had teaching duties from 1768 at St. George's Hospital, to which he had been elected surgeon in 1758. In 1760 Hunter accepted a commission as an army surgeon. He returned to London in 1763, where he continued in private practice until his death. In 1776 he was named surgeon extraordinary to King George III.

Hunter not only made specific contributions of great importance in surgery but also attained for surgery the dignity of a scientific profession, basing its practice on a vast body of general biological principles. In an attempt to demonstrate that gonorrhea and syphilis are manifestations of a single disease, he inoculated a subject (sometimes said to have been himself) with pus from a person with gonorrhea. The subject developed symptoms of both diseases.

Hunter wrote *The Natural History of the Human Teeth* (1771), *A Treatise on the Venereal Disease* (1786), and *Observations on Certain Parts of the Animal Oeconomy* (1786). *A Treatise on the Blood, Inflammation, and Gun-shot Wounds* was published posthumously in 1794. Hunter's vast collection of anatomical and pathological specimens was bought by Parliament for the Royal College of Surgeons in 1799.

WILLIAM WITHERING
(born March 17, 1741, Wellington, Shropshire, England–died Oct. 6, 1799, Sparkbrook, Birmingham, Warwickshire)

William Withering was an English physician best known for his use of extracts of foxglove (*Digitalis purpurea*) to treat dropsy (edema), a condition associated with heart failure and characterized by the accumulation of fluid in soft tissues. Withering's insights on the medical uses of foxglove proved crucial to modern understanding of heart failure, and today drugs containing the active compound, known as digitalis, are still prescribed.

Education and Early Career in Medicine

Influenced by his father, Edmund, who worked as an apothecary, and by his uncle, Brooke Hector, who worked as a physician in Lichfield, Withering enrolled at the University of Edinburgh in 1762, following four years of medical apprenticeship. In 1766, having shown little interest in botany, which formed a large part of the medical curriculum at the time, he prepared his thesis on malignant sore throat, titled *De Angina Gangraenosa*. This was also the year that—following a thorough self-study of the Bible and sacred history—Withering changed from an atheist to a Christian. While in Edinburgh, he also participated in Masonic activities.

Withering soon relocated to Stafford, where he attended private patients and served as a founding physician of the Stafford General Infirmary. He began to enjoy botany and met Helena Cookes, who sketched the plants he collected. They were married on Sept. 12, 1772, and had three children. Seeking a more substantial income, Withering decided to move to Birmingham to fill a vacancy created by the death of physician and Lunar Society cofounder William Small in 1775. (The Lunar Society was a gathering of naturalists and inventors who met monthly in the Midlands of England, traveling under the light of the full moon.) The move to Birmingham was suggested to Withering by Lichfield physician Erasmus Darwin. Together with fellow physician John Ash, Withering served as a founder of the Birmingham General Hospital, which opened in 1779. There he treated several thousand patients each year, many of whom were impoverished and received their care gratis.

Botanical Works

Withering's lasting reputation lies primarily with his publication *An Account of the Foxglove, and Some of Its Medical Uses* (1785). Though foxglove (*Digitalis purpurea*) had been used in folk medicine for centuries, Withering drew upon 156 of his own cases to objectively demonstrate its efficacy in treating dropsy, an abnormal accumulation of watery fluid in the intercellular spaces of connective tissue that typically accompanied heart failure. In particular, he noted that foxglove leaf preparations were efficacious in small, nontoxic doses and that their action varied according to the plant's stage of bloom. Withering's publication created considerable furor with fellow Lunar Society member Erasmus Darwin, who claimed priority in having published on foxglove's therapeutic use in managing dropsy. This was not the first conflict between Withering and Darwin. The previous year, Darwin, together with fellow members of the Lichfield Botanical Society, had published the first English translation of Swedish naturalist and explorer Carolus Linnaeus's *Genera et Species Plantarum* (the translated text was published in 1784) without acknowledging Withering's contributions.

Withering gained renown for his botanical writings, the first of which, following in the tradition of English naturalist John Ray, was *A Botanical Arrangement of All the Vegetables Growing Naturally in G. Britain* (1776). Withering's later work, *An Arrangement of British Plants* (1787–92), was designed to show amateur botanists, many of whom were young women, the utility of the Linnaean classification system (which introduced the standard hierarchy of class, order, genus, and species and provided workable keys, making it possible to identify plants and animals from Linnaeus's books). In addition, this work introduced Withering's specially designed field microscope, which subsequently became known as the Withering botanical microscope.

Influence on Medicine and Science

Withering contributed to the clinical distinction of scarlet fever and to the medical use of lead and rum. Following the Birmingham riots of 1791, he left England and went to Portugal, where, as he had done in Stafford and Birmingham, he analyzed the mineral content of spa waters. In 1783 he prepared the English translation of Swedish chemist and naturalist Torbern Bergman's mineralogy treatise, and, in recognition for his study of the properties of barium carbonate, this mineral was subsequently named witherite. The flowering plant *Witheringia solanacea* (order Solanales) was also named in his honour.

In 1794 Withering returned to Birmingham, where he died following complications of tuberculosis. He was buried at Edgbaston Old Church in Edgbaston, Birmingham, where his memorial tablet is marked by the staff and snake of Asclepius, the Greco-Roman god of medicine, and sprigs of *Digitalis* and *Witheringia*. Today digitalis continues to serve as the active ingredient of the cardiac glycoside drugs digoxin and digitoxin.

BENJAMIN RUSH
(born Jan. 4, 1746, [Dec. 24, 1745, Old Style], Byberry, near Philadelphia, Pa., U.S.–died April 19, 1813, Philadelphia)

Benjamin Rush was an American physician and political leader, a member of the Continental Congress and a signer of the Declaration of Independence. His encouragement of clinical research and instruction was frequently offset by his insistence upon bloodletting, purging, and other debilitating therapeutic measures.

Rush was born into a pious Presbyterian family. He was sent to a private academy and on to the College of New Jersey at Princeton, from which he was graduated in 1760. After a medical apprenticeship of six years, he sailed for Europe. He took a medical degree at the University of Edinburgh in 1768 and then worked in London hospitals and briefly visited Paris.

Returning home to begin medical practice in 1769, he was appointed professor of chemistry at the College of Philadelphia, and in the following year he published his *Syllabus of a Course of Lectures on Chemistry,* the first American textbook in this field. Despite war and political upheavals, Rush's practice grew to substantial proportions, partly owing to his literary output. The standard checklist of early American medical imprints lists 65 publications under his name, not counting scores of communications to newspapers and magazines. Another source of Rush's professional prestige was the large number of his private apprentices and students from all over the country. He taught some 3,000 students during his tenure as professor of, successively, chemistry, the theory and practice of medicine, and the institutes of medicine and clinical medicine at the College of Philadelphia and the University of Pennsylvania. After 1790 his lectures were among the leading cultural attractions of the city.

As a physician, Rush was a theorist, and a dogmatic one, rather than a scientific pathologist. Striving for a simple, unitary explanation of disease, he conjectured that all diseases are really one—a fever brought on by overstimulation of the blood vessels—and hence subject to a simple remedy—"depletion" by bloodletting and purges. The worse the fever, he believed, the more "heroic" the treatment it called for; in the epidemics of yellow fever that afflicted Philadelphia in the 1790s his cures were more dreaded by some than the disease.

In psychiatry Rush's contributions were more enduring. For many years he laboured among the insane patients at the Pennsylvania Hospital, advocating humane treatment for them on the ground that mental disorders were as subject to healing arts as physical ones; indeed, he held that insanity often proceeded from physical causes, an idea that was a long step forward from the old notion that lunatics are possessed by devils. However, he also advocated for some harsher methods, including the practice of restraining mental patients with his notorious "tranquilising chair." Still, his *Medical Inquiries and Observations upon the Diseases of the Mind,* published in 1812, was the first and for many years the only American treatise on psychiatry.

Rush was an early and active American patriot. As a member of the radical provincial conference in June 1776, he drafted a resolution urging independence and was soon elected to the Continental Congress, signing the Declaration of Independence with other members on August 2. For a year he served in the field as surgeon general and physician general of the Middle Department of the Continental Army, but early in 1778 he resigned because he considered the military hospitals mismanaged by his superior, who was supported by General Washington. Rush went on to question Washington's military judgment, a step that he was to regret and one that clouded his reputation until recent times. He resumed the practice and teaching of medicine and in 1797, by appointment of Pres. John Adams, took on the duties of treasurer of the U.S. Mint. He held this office until his death.

EDWARD JENNER

(born May 17, 1749, Berkeley, Gloucestershire, England–died Jan. 26, 1823, Berkeley)

Edward Jenner was an English surgeon who was best known as the discoverer of vaccination for smallpox. Jenner was born at a time when the patterns of British medical practice and education were undergoing gradual change. Slowly the division between the Oxford- or Cambridge-trained physicians and the apothecaries or surgeons—who were much less educated and who acquired their medical knowledge through apprenticeship rather than through academic work—was becoming less sharp, and hospital work was becoming much more important.

Jenner was a country youth, the son of a clergyman. Because Edward was only five when his father died, he was brought up by an older brother, who was also a clergyman. Edward acquired a love of nature that remained with him all his life. He attended grammar school and at the age of 13 was apprenticed to a nearby surgeon. In the following eight years Jenner acquired a sound knowledge of medical and surgical practice. On completing his apprenticeship at the age of 21, he went to London and became the house pupil of John Hunter, who was on the staff of St. George's Hospital and was one of the most prominent surgeons in London. Even more important, however, he was an anatomist, biologist, and experimentalist of the first rank; not only did he collect biological specimens, but he also concerned himself with problems of physiology and function.

The firm friendship that grew between the two men lasted until Hunter's death in 1793. From no one else could Jenner have received the stimuli that so confirmed his natural bent—a catholic interest in biological phenomena, disciplined powers of observation, sharpening of critical faculties, and a reliance on experimental investigation. From Hunter, Jenner received the characteristic advice, "Why think [i.e., speculate]—why not try the experiment?"

In addition to his training and experience in biology, Jenner made progress in clinical surgery. After studying in London from 1770 to 1773, he returned to country practice in Berkeley and enjoyed substantial success. He was capable, skillful, and popular. In addition to practicing medicine, he joined two medical groups for the promotion of medical knowledge and wrote occasional medical papers. He played the violin in a musical club, wrote light verse, and, as a naturalist, made many observations, particularly on the nesting habits of the cuckoo and on bird migration. He also collected specimens for Hunter; many of Hunter's letters to Jenner have been preserved, but Jenner's letters to Hunter have unfortunately been lost. After one disappointment in love in 1778, Jenner married in 1788.

Smallpox was widespread in the 18th century, and occasional outbreaks of special intensity resulted in a very high death rate. Smallpox begins with a high fever, headache, and back pain and then proceeds to an eruption on the skin that leaves the face and limbs covered with cratered pockmarks, or pox. For centuries smallpox was one of the world's most dreaded plagues, killing as many as 30 percent of its victims, most of them children. The disease, a leading cause of death at the time, respected no social class, and disfigurement, and sometimes blindness, were not uncommon in patients who recovered.

The only means of combating smallpox was a primitive form of vaccination called variolation—intentionally infecting a healthy person with the "matter" taken from a patient sick with a mild attack of the disease. The practice, which originated in China and India, was based on two distinct concepts: first, that one attack of smallpox effectively protected against any subsequent attack and, second, that a person deliberately infected with a mild case of the disease would safely acquire such protection. It was, in present-day terminology, an "elective" infection—i.e., one given to a person in good health. Unfortunately, the transmitted disease did not always remain mild, and mortality sometimes occurred. Furthermore, the inoculated person could disseminate the disease to others and thus act as a focus of infection.

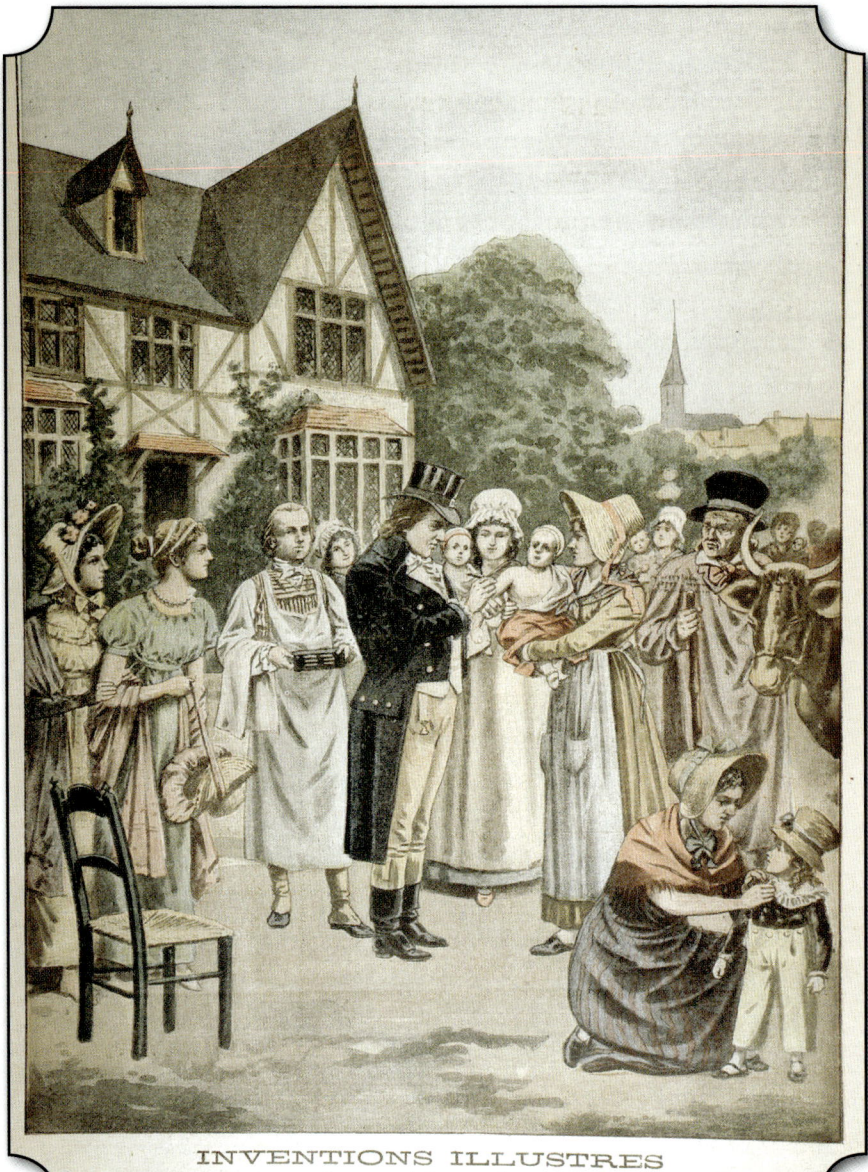

In this rendering, Edward Jenner uses cowpox serum to vaccinate a small boy against smallpox.

Jenner had been impressed by the fact that a person who had suffered an attack of cowpox—a relatively harmless disease that could be contracted from cattle—could not take the smallpox—i.e., could not become infected whether by accidental or intentional exposure to smallpox. Pondering this phenomenon, Jenner concluded that cowpox not only protected against smallpox but could be transmitted from one person to another as a deliberate mechanism of protection.

The story of the great breakthrough is well known. In May 1796 Jenner found a young dairymaid, Sarah Nelmes, who had fresh cowpox lesions on her hand. On May 14, using matter from Sarah's lesions, he inoculated an eight-year-old boy, James Phipps, who had never had smallpox. Phipps became slightly ill over the course of the next 9 days but was well on the 10th. On July 1 Jenner inoculated the boy again, this time with smallpox matter. No disease developed; protection was complete. In 1798 Jenner, having added further cases, published privately a slender book entitled *An Inquiry into the Causes and Effects of the Variolae Vaccinae*.

The reaction to the publication was not immediately favourable. Jenner went to London seeking volunteers for vaccination but, in a stay of three months, was not successful. In London vaccination became popularized through the activities of others, particularly the surgeon Henry Cline, to whom Jenner had given some of the inoculant, and the doctors George Pearson and William Woodville. Difficulties arose, some of them quite unpleasant; Pearson tried to take credit away from Jenner, and Woodville, a physician in a smallpox hospital, contaminated the cowpox matter with smallpox virus. Vaccination rapidly proved its value, however, and Jenner became intensely active promoting it. The procedure spread rapidly to America and the rest of Europe and soon was carried around the world.

Complications were many. Vaccination seemed simple, but the vast number of persons who practiced it did not necessarily follow the procedure that Jenner had recommended, and deliberate or unconscious innovations often impaired the effectiveness. Pure cowpox vaccine was not always easy to obtain, nor was it easy to preserve or transmit. Furthermore, the biological factors that produce immunity were not yet understood; much information had to be gathered and a great many mistakes made before a fully effective procedure could be developed, even on an empirical basis.

Despite errors and occasional chicanery, the death rate from smallpox plunged. Jenner received worldwide recognition and many honours, but he made no attempt to enrich himself through his discovery and actually devoted so much time to the cause of vaccination that his private practice and personal affairs suffered severely. Parliament voted him a sum of £10,000 in 1802 and a further sum of £20,000 in 1806. Jenner not only received honours but also aroused opposition and found himself subjected to attacks and calumnies, despite which he continued his activities on behalf of vaccination. His wife, ill with tuberculosis, died in 1815, and Jenner retired from public life. It took almost another half century to discover an effective method of producing antiviral vaccines that were both safe and effective.

RENÉ-THÉOPHILE-HYACINTHE LAËNNEC

(born Feb. 17, 1781, Quimper, Brittany, France–died Aug. 13, 1826, Kerlouanec)

René-Théophile-Hyacinthe Laënnec was a French physician who invented the stethoscope and perfected the art of auditory examination of the chest cavity.

When Laënnec was five years old, his mother, Michelle Félicité Guesdon, died from tuberculosis, leaving Laënnec and his brother, Michaud, in the incompetent care of their father, Théophile-Marie Laënnec, who worked as a civil servant and had a reputation for reckless spending. In 1793, during the French Revolution, Laënnec went to live with his uncle, Guillaume-François Laënnec, in the port city of Nantes, located in the Pays de la Loire region of western France. Laënnec's uncle was the dean of medicine at the University of Nantes. Although the region was in the midst of counterrevolutionary revolts, the young Laënnec settled into his academic training and, under his uncle's direction, began his medical studies. His first experience working in a hospital setting was at the Hôtel-Dieu of Nantes, where he learned to apply surgical dressings and to care for patients. In 1800 Laënnec went to Paris and entered the École Pratique, studying anatomy and dissection in the laboratory of surgeon and pathologist Guillaume Dupuytren. Dupuytren was a bright and ambitious academic who became known for his many surgical accomplishments and for his work in alleviating permanent tissue contracture in the palm, a condition later named Dupuytren contracture. While Dupuytren undoubtedly influenced Laënnec's studies, Laënnec also received instruction from other well-known French anatomists and physicians, including Gaspard Laurent Bayle, who studied tuberculosis and cancer; Marie-François-Xavier Bichat, who helped establish histology, the study of tissues; and Jean-Nicolas Corvisart des Marets, who used chest percussion to assess heart function and who served as personal physician to Napoleon I.

Laënnec became known for his studies of peritonitis (inflammation of the peritoneum, the membrane that lines the abdominal wall and then folds in to enclose the abdominal organs), amenorrhea (failure to menstruate), the prostate gland, and tubercle lesions. He graduated in 1804 and continued his research as a faculty member of the Society of the School of Medicine in Paris. He wrote several articles on pathological anatomy and became devoted to Roman Catholicism, which led to his appointment as personal physician to Joseph Cardinal Fesch, half brother of Napoleon and French ambassador to the Vatican in Rome. Laënnec remained Fesch's physician until 1814, when the cardinal was exiled after Napoleon's empire fell.

While Laënnec's embrace of Catholic doctrine was viewed favourably by royalists, many in the medical profession criticized his conservatism, which contradicted the views of many academicians. Nonetheless, Laënnec's restored faith inspired him to find better ways to care for people, especially the poor. From 1812 to 1813, during the Napoleonic Wars, Laënnec took charge of the wards in the Salpêtrière Hospital in Paris, which was reserved for wounded soldiers. After the return of the monarchy, in 1816 Laënnec was appointed as physician at the Necker Hospital in Paris, where he developed the stethoscope.

Laënnec's original stethoscope design consisted of a hollow tube of wood that was 3.5 cm (1.4 inches) in diameter and 25 cm (10 inches) long and was monoaural, transmitting sound to one ear. It could be easily disassembled and reassembled, and it used a special plug to facilitate the transmission of sounds from the patient's heart and lungs. His instrument replaced the practice of immediate auscultation, in which the physician laid his ear on the chest of the patient to listen to chest sounds. The awkwardness that this method created in the case of women patients compelled Laënnec to find a better way to listen to the chest. His wooden monoaural stethoscope was replaced by models using rubber tubing at the end of the 19th century. Other advancements include the development of binaural stethoscopes, capable of transmitting sounds to both ears of the physician.

In 1819 Laënnec published *De l'auscultation médiate* ("On Mediate Auscultation"), the first discourse on a variety of heart and lung sounds heard through the stethoscope. The first English translation of *De l'auscultation médiate* was published in London in 1821. Laënnec's treatise aroused intense interest, and physicians from throughout Europe came to Paris to learn about Laënnec's diagnostic tool. He became an internationally renowned lecturer. In 1822 Laënnec was appointed chair and professor of medicine at the College of France, and the following year he became a full member of the French Academy of Medicine and a professor at the medical clinic of the Charity Hospital in Paris. In 1824 he was made a chevalier of the Legion of Honour. That same year Laënnec married Jacquette Guichard, a widow. They did not have any children, his wife having suffered a miscarriage. Two years later at the age of 45 Laënnec died from cavitating tuberculosis—the same disease that he helped elucidate using his stethoscope. Using his own invention, he could diagnose himself and understand that he was dying.

Because Laënnec's stethoscope enabled heart and lung sounds to be heard without placing an ear on the patient's chest, the stethoscope technique became known as the "mediate" method for auscultation. Throughout Laënnec's medical work and research, his diagnoses were supported with observations and findings from autopsies. In addition to revolutionizing the diagnosis of lung disorders, Laënnec introduced many terms still used today. For example, *Laënnec's cirrhosis*, used to describe micronodular cirrhosis (growth of small masses of tissue in the liver that cause degeneration of liver function), and *melanose* (Greek, meaning "black"), which he coined in 1804 to describe melanoma. Laënnec was the first to recognize that melanotic lesions were the result of metastatic melanoma, in which cancer cells from the original tumour site spread to other organs and tissues in the body. He is considered the father of clinical auscultation, and he wrote the first descriptions of pneumonia, bronchiectasis, pleurisy, emphysema, and pneumothorax. His classification of pulmonary conditions is still used today.

FRANÇOIS MAGENDIE
(born Oct. 6, 1783, Bordeaux, France–died Oct. 7, 1855, Sannois)

François Magendie was a French experimental physiologist who was the first to prove the functional difference of the spinal nerves. His pioneer studies of the effects of drugs on various parts of the body led to the scientific introduction into medical practice of such compounds as strychnine and morphine. In 1822 he confirmed and elaborated the observation by the Scottish anatomist Sir Charles Bell (1811) that the anterior roots of the spinal nerves are motor in function, while the posterior roots serve to communicate sensory impulses.

Appointed professor of medicine at the Collège de France, Paris (1831), Magendie was one of the first to observe anaphylaxis (an exaggerated reaction by an animal to the injection into its blood of a foreign protein) when he found (1839) that rabbits able to tolerate a single injection of egg albumin often died following a second injection. Founder of the first periodical of experimental physiology, *Journal de Physiologie Expérimentale* (1821), Magendie greatly influenced the intellectual development of the renowned French physiologist Claude Bernard, one of his students (1841–43). Magendie was elected to the French Academy of Sciences in 1821 and served as its president in 1837.

JOHN SNOW

(born March 15, 1813, York, Yorkshire, England–died June 16, 1858, London)

John Snow was an English physician known for his seminal studies of cholera and widely viewed as the father of contemporary epidemiology. His best-known studies include his investigation of London's Broad Street pump outbreak, which occurred in 1854, and his "Grand Experiment," a study comparing waterborne cholera cases in two regions of the city—one receiving sewage-contaminated water and the other receiving relatively clean water. Snow's innovative reasoning and approach to the control of this deadly disease remain valid and are considered exemplary for epidemiologists throughout the world. Snow's reputation in anesthesiology, specifically in regard to his knowledge of ether and chloroform, was considerable, such that he was asked to administer chloroform to Queen Victoria when she gave birth in 1853 to Prince Leopold and in 1857 to Princess Beatrice. Snow's achievements are considered remarkable, given his humble origin and short life; a stroke caused his death at age 45.

EDUCATION AND CONTRIBUTIONS TO ANESTHESIOLOGY

Snow was born in York, England, where his father worked as a labourer in a coal yard. He was the firstborn in a family of nine children. At age 14, after spending his early years at a school in York, he left home and pursued three consecutive medical apprenticeships in various regions of Yorkshire. In 1831, when visiting coal miners, he had his first encounter with cholera, a disease that would later become the focus of his scientific endeavours. By 1836 Snow had begun his formal medical education, eventually receiving a doctor of medicine degree (1844) from the University of London. In 1849 he became a licentiate (licensed specialist) of the Royal College of Physicians of London, rising to an elite level in the medical profession. He lived, conducted research, and maintained a medical practice in the Soho neighbourhood of London.

In 1846 Snow learned of the use of ether in America to relieve pain during surgery. He soon mastered its use, and in 1847 he was appointed as anesthesiologist at St. George's Hospital. Later that year he started working with chloroform. Finding the prevailing drops-in-handkerchief method to be too crude, he developed an apparatus that improved both the safety and the effectiveness of chloroform. His success with administering chloroform to Queen Victoria produced a dramatic increase in the social acceptance of gaseous anesthesia. Snow spoke extensively on his work with anesthetics and wrote the influential book *On Chloroform and Other Anaesthetics*, which was published shortly after his death in 1858.

Broad Street Pump and the "Grand Experiment"

Many British physicians investigated the epidemiology of cholera. Cholera, an acute infection of the small intestine, is caused by the bacterium *Vibrio cholerae* and characterized by extreme diarrhea with rapid and severe depletion of body fluids and salts. Cholera is a disease that can incite populations to panic. Its reputation as a fierce and unrelenting killer is a deserved one.

The first cholera epidemic in London occurred in 1831–32, when Snow was still learning his craft. When the second cholera epidemic occurred, in 1848–49, he and others founded the London Epidemiological Society, intending to advise the government on ways to combat the disease. Snow reasoned that cholera was caused by a microbelike agent, or germ, that was spread through direct fecal contact, contaminated water, and soiled clothing. However, his theory was at odds with the then prevailing theory that cholera was spread by bad air, or miasma, arising from decayed organic matter. The two etiologic hypotheses—germ theory and miasma—were widely debated, with available clinical and population-based evidence serving as the basis for arguments from both sides. The etiologic debate raged for many years. It was not until the causative organism, *Vibrio cholerae* (initially discovered in 1854), was well characterized in the 1880s that the debate was decided in favour of germ theory.

Snow's respected reputation in epidemiology arose from two classic studies of the third epidemic to reach England, which began in 1853 and lasted until 1855. The first study concerned the Broad Street pump outbreak of 1854, which killed many persons in the Soho neighbourhood. He used skilled reasoning, graphs, and maps to demonstrate the impact of the contaminated water coming from the Broad Street pump. He informed the local authorities and explained his hunch as to the cause. Although the authorities were skeptical, the next day they had the pump disabled by removing its handle. Almost immediately, new cases of cholera started to dwindle. However, because cholera deaths were already declining in the city, Snow was unable to attribute the end of the outbreak directly to the removal of the pump handle.

The second study was the "Grand Experiment," also of 1854, which compared London neighbourhoods receiving water from two different companies. The

Southwark and Vauxhall Company drew its water from sewage-polluted inlets of the River Thames in London, whereas the Lambeth Company obtained its water from the upper portion of the river, some distance from urban pollution. Snow showed that cholera deaths were higher for residents in homes served by the Southwark and Vauxhall Company than for residents in locations served by the Lambeth Company. Snow showed the harmful effect of contaminated water in two nearly equivalent populations, and he suggested intervention strategies to control the epidemic. His ideas and observations, including innovative disease maps, were published in his book *On the Mode of Communication of Cholera* (1855). Later, in the 1930s, Snow's work was republished as a classic work in epidemiology, resulting in lasting recognition of his work.

ANN PRESTON

(born Dec. 1, 1813, West Grove, Pa., U.S.–died April 18, 1872, Philadelphia)

Ann Preston was an American physician and educator who struggled for the rights of women to learn, practice, and teach medicine in the mid-1800s. Preston was educated in Quaker schools and later became active in the abolition and temperance movements. Her temperance work had aroused in her an interest in physiology and hygiene, and she studied those subjects as well as Latin on her own for a time. She began to teach classes in physiology and hygiene to other interested women and in 1847 became a medical apprentice in the office of a physician friend in Philadelphia. Two years later, having completed her apprenticeship, Preston was refused admission to all four Philadelphia medical colleges because of her sex. In October 1850, however, she entered the newly established Female (later Woman's) Medical College of Pennsylvania with the first class, and she graduated in 1851. After further study she was appointed professor of physiology and hygiene at the college in 1853.

In 1858 the Board of Censors of the Philadelphia Medical Society effectively banned women physicians from the public teaching clinics of the city. In order to provide vital clinical experience to the college's students, Preston began raising funds for a women's hospital to be affiliated with the college. A board of women managers, of which she was a member, was appointed to direct the planning and operation of the hospital. The college closed on the outbreak of the Civil War in 1861, but the Woman's Hospital opened later that year. The Woman's Medical College, operating under a new charter, opened the following year. In 1863 Preston worked with Emeline H. Cleveland, chief resident of Woman's Hospital, to establish a training school for nurses, and in 1866 Preston was chosen first woman dean of the college. She continued in that post as well as in her professorship for the rest of her life.

Under Preston's leadership the students of the Woman's Medical College were at last admitted to the leading general clinics in Philadelphia in 1868. The

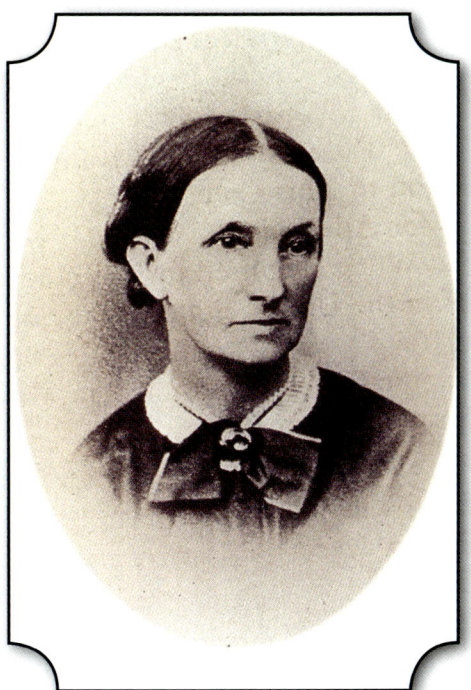

Ann Preston helped improve women's access to quality medical education.

following year, in response to a remonstrance by other local medical colleges and hospitals and numerous individual doctors, she published in the Philadelphia newspapers a classic argument in support of women physicians.

HORACE WELLS

(born Jan. 21, 1815, Hartford, Vt., U.S.–died Jan. 24, 1848, New York, N.Y.)

Horace Wells, an American dentist, was a pioneer in the use of surgical anesthesia. Drugs of various kinds have been used for many centuries to reduce the distress of surgical operations. Homer wrote of nepenthe, which was probably cannabis or opium. Arabian physicians used opium and henbane. Centuries later, powerful rum was administered freely to British sailors before emergency amputations were carried out on board ship in the aftermath of battle.

In 1799 Sir Humphry Davy, British chemist and inventor, tried inhaling nitrous oxide ("laughing gas") and discovered its anesthetic properties, but the implications of his findings for surgery were ignored. By the early 1840s parties had become fashionable in Britain and the United States at which nitrous oxide, contained in bladders, was passed around and inhaled for its soporific effect. It was soon found that ether, which could be carried much more conveniently in small bottles, was equally potent. In the United States several young dentists and doctors experimented independently with the use of nitrous oxide or ether to dull the pain of tooth extractions and other minor operations.

While practicing in Hartford, Conn., in 1844, Wells noted the pain-killing properties of nitrous oxide during a laughing-gas road show and thereafter used it in performing painless dental operations. He was allowed to demonstrate the method at the Massachusetts General Hospital in January 1845, but when the patient proved unresponsive to the gas, Wells was exposed to ridicule.

After William Morton, a dental surgeon and Wells's former partner, successfully demonstrated ether anesthesia in October 1846, Wells began extensive self-experimentation with nitrous oxide, ether, chloroform, and other chemicals to ascertain their comparative anesthetic properties. His personality radically altered by frequent inhalation of chemical vapours, he was jailed in New York City for throwing acid at passersby. There, in a jail cell, he took his own life while the Paris Medical Society was publicly acclaiming him the discoverer of anesthetic gases.

IGNAZ PHILIPP SEMMELWEIS
(born July 1, 1818, Buda, Hungary, Austrian Empire [now Budapest, Hungary]–died Aug. 13, 1865, Vienna, Austria)

Ignaz Philipp Semmelweis (Hungarian Ignác Fülöp Semmelweis) was a German Hungarian physician who discovered the cause of puerperal (childbed) fever and introduced antisepsis (the inhibiting of the growth and multiplication of microorganisms by any of several substances) into medical practice.

Educated at the universities of Pest and Vienna, Semmelweis received his doctor's degree from Vienna in 1844 and was appointed assistant at the obstetric clinic in Vienna. He soon became involved in the problem of puerperal infection, the scourge of maternity hospitals throughout Europe. The infection of some part of the female reproductive organs follows childbirth or abortion. The infection is most commonly of the raw surface of the interior of the uterus after separation of the placenta (afterbirth), but pathogenic organisms may also affect lacerations of any part of the genital tract. By whatever portal, they can invade the bloodstream and lymph system to cause septicemia (blood poisoning), cellulitis (inflammation of cellular tissue), and pelvic or generalized peritonitis (inflammation of the abdominal lining). The severity of the illness depends on the virulence of the infecting organism, the resistance of the invaded tissues, and the general health of the patient. Abortions performed in unhygienic surroundings commonly result in puerperal fever.

Although most women delivered at home, those who had to seek hospitalization because of poverty, illegitimacy, or obstetrical complications faced mortality rates ranging as high as 25–30 percent. Some thought that the infection was induced by overcrowding, poor ventilation, the onset of lactation, or miasma. Semmelweis proceeded to investigate its cause over the strong objections of his chief, who, like other continental physicians, had reconciled himself to the idea that the disease was unpreventable.

Semmelweis observed that, among women in the first division of the clinic, the death rate from childbed fever was two or three times as high as among those in the second division, although the two divisions were identical with the exception that students were taught in the first and midwives in the second. He put forward the thesis that perhaps the students carried something to the patients they examined during labour. The death of a friend from a wound infection incurred during the examination of a woman who died of puerperal infection and the similarity of the findings in the two cases gave support to his reasoning. He concluded that students who came directly from the dissecting room to the maternity ward carried the infection from mothers who had died of the disease to healthy mothers. He ordered the students to wash their hands in a solution of chlorinated lime before each examination.

Under these procedures, the mortality rates in the first division dropped from 18.27 to 1.27 percent, and in March and August of 1848 no woman died in childbirth in his division. The younger medical men in Vienna recognized the significance of Semmelweis's discovery and gave him all possible assistance. His superior, on the other hand, was critical—not because he wanted to oppose him but because he failed to understand him.

In the year 1848 a liberal political revolution swept Europe, and Semmelweis took part in the events in Vienna. After the revolution had been put down, Semmelweis found that his political activities had increased the obstacles to his professional work. In 1849 he was dropped from his post at the clinic. He then applied for a teaching post at the university in midwifery but was turned down. Soon after that, he gave a successful lecture at the Medical Society of Vienna entitled "The Origin of Puerperal Fever." At the same time, he applied once more for the teaching post, but, although he received it, there were restrictions attached to it that he considered humiliating. He left Vienna and returned to Pest in 1850.

He worked for the next six years at the St. Rochus Hospital in Pest. An epidemic of puerperal fever had broken out in the obstetrics department, and, at his request, Semmelweis was put in charge of the department. His measures promptly reduced the mortality rate, and in his years there it averaged only 0.85 percent. In Prague and Vienna, meantime, the rate was still from 10 to 15 percent.

In 1855 he was appointed professor of obstetrics at the University of Pest. He married, had five children, and developed his private practice. His ideas were accepted in Hungary, and the government addressed a circular to all district authorities ordering the introduction of the prophylactic methods of Semmelweis. In 1857 he declined the chair of obstetrics at the University of Zürich. Vienna remained hostile toward him, and the editor of the *Wiener Medizinische Wochenschrift* wrote that it was time to stop the nonsense about the chlorine hand wash.

In 1861 Semmelweis published his principal work, *Die Ätiologie, der Begriff und die Prophylaxis des Kindbettfiebers* (*The Etiology, Concept, and Prophylaxis of Childbed Fever*). He sent it to all the prominent obstetricians and medical societies abroad, but the general reaction was adverse. The weight of authority stood against his teachings. He addressed several open letters to professors of medicine in other countries, but to little effect. At a conference of German physicians and natural scientists, most of the speakers—including the pathologist Rudolf Virchow—rejected his doctrine. The years of controversy gradually undermined his spirit. In 1865 he suffered a breakdown and was taken to a mental hospital, where he died. Ironically, his illness and death were caused by the infection of a wound on his right hand, apparently the result of an operation he had performed before being taken ill. He died of the same disease against which he had struggled all his professional life.

Semmelweis's doctrine was subsequently accepted by medical science. His influence on the development of knowledge and control of infection was hailed by Joseph Lister, the father of modern antisepsis: "I think with the greatest admiration of him and his achievement and it fills me with joy that at last he is given the respect due to him."

MAYO FAMILY

William Worrall Mayo (born May 31, 1819, near Manchester, England—died March 6, 1911, Rochester, Minn., U.S.)
William James Mayo (born June 29, 1861, Le Sueur, Minn., U.S.—died July 28, 1939, Rochester, Minn.)
Charles Horace Mayo (born July 19, 1865, Rochester, Minn., U.S.— died May 26, 1939, Chicago, Ill.)
Charles William Mayo (born July 28, 1898, Rochester, Minn., U.S.—d. July 28, 1968, Rochester)

The Mayo family is perhaps the most famous group of physicians in the United States. Three generations of the Mayo family established at Rochester, Minn., the world-renowned nonprofit Mayo Clinic and the Mayo Foundation for Medical Education and Research, which are dedicated to diagnosing and treating nearly every known illness.

William Worrall Mayo was the father of the doctors Mayo who developed a large-scale practice of medicine. Mayo studied chemistry at Owens College in Manchester and, after immigrating to the United States in 1845, learned medicine from a private physician in Lafayette, Ind., subsequently receiving degrees from Indiana Medical College, La Porte, and the University of Missouri, Columbia. In 1863 he moved to Rochester, where he soon had an extensive surgical practice. After taking care of the casualties of a disastrous tornado in Rochester, with the assistance of the Sisters of St. Francis, Mayo, his two sons, and the sisters planned to erect a new hospital. St. Mary's Hospital was opened on Oct. 1, 1889, and Mayo and his two sons became responsible for care of the patients. After the father retired, the work at the hospital was continued by his sons.

William James Mayo was the eldest son of William Worrall Mayo. He received his M.D. degree in 1883 from the University of Michigan, Ann Arbor, and then engaged at Rochester in the private practice of medicine and surgery with his father and later with his younger brother Charles Horace Mayo. Though William J. Mayo became the administrator in the practice, no important decisions were made without the full agreement of both brothers. He and his brother performed all the surgeries at St. Mary's Hospital until about 1905. From this surgical partnership of the two brothers evolved the cooperative group clinic, later known as the Mayo Clinic. William James Mayo, who became a specialist in surgery of the abdomen, pelvis, and kidney, remained active in surgery at the clinic until 1928 and in administration until 1933.

Charles Horace Mayo, the younger son of William Worrall Mayo, was characterized as a "surgical wonder." He received an M.D. degree from the Chicago Medical College (later part of Northwestern University Medical School) in 1888 and in the same year began private practice of surgery with his father and brother.

Charles Mayo had the ability to work in all surgical fields; he originated modern procedures in goitre surgery and in neurosurgery; he performed highly successful operations for cataract of the eye and originated procedures for several orthopedic operations. In 1930 he retired from surgery at the clinic and three years later from administration. He was professor of surgery at the University of Minnesota Medical School from 1919 to 1936 and at the University of Minnesota Graduate School from 1915 to 1936. In regard to his brother, William J. Mayo said, "Charlie has...an intuitive mind, from his knowledge of physiology and anatomy and his understanding of the personality of the patient." At one time he was a member of the advisory board of *Encyclopædia Britannica*. With his brother, he alternated as chief consultant for all surgical services in the U.S. Army during World War I, serving with the rank of colonel. After the war, each brother was commissioned a brigadier general in the medical-corps reserve.

Charles William Mayo was the son of Charles Horace. He was a skilled surgeon and member of the board of governors of the Mayo Clinic, chairman of the Mayo Association, and a member (chairman 1961–67) of the board of regents of the University of Minnesota. He is noted for a speech he gave in 1953 as a member of the United States delegation at the United Nations.

The clinic began to grow in size in the early 1900s, when many young physicians began to apply for positions as interns and assistants. At the same time, outstanding scientists in basic medical subjects were added to the clinic's training and research programs. In 1919 the Mayo brothers transferred property and capital to the Mayo Properties Association, later called the Mayo Foundation, a charitable and educational corporation having a perpetual charter. About 1900 the Mayo Clinic was changed from a partnership to a voluntary association of physicians and specialists in allied fields.

In 1915 the Mayo brothers gave $1.5 million to the University of Minnesota to establish the Mayo Foundation for Medical Education and Research at Rochester in connection with the clinic. The foundation, which is part of the University of Minnesota Graduate School, offers graduate training in medicine and related subjects.

In 1986 the Mayo Clinic merged with the nearby St. Mary's Hospital and Rochester Methodist Hospital. The Mayo Foundation also began a national expansion program that year, opening the Mayo Clinic Jacksonville in Florida; the Mayo Clinic Scottsdale in Arizona opened in 1987. In 1992 the Mayo Foundation launched the Mayo Health System, a network of clinics, hospitals, and health-care facilities (including nursing homes) serving communities in Iowa, Minnesota, and Wisconsin.

By 2015, the Mayo Clinic's three sites employed more than 4,200 physicians, researchers, and scientists and more than 52,900 allied health staff and treated more than one million patients annually. The clinic produces several publications, including *Mayo Magazine*.

WILLIAM THOMAS GREEN MORTON
(born Aug. 9, 1819, Charlton, Mass., U.S.–died July 15, 1868, New York, N.Y.)

William Thomas Green Morton was an American dental surgeon who in 1846 gave the first successful public demonstration of ether anesthesia during surgery. He is credited with gaining the medical world's acceptance of surgical anesthesia.

Morton began dental practice in Boston in 1844. In January 1845 he was present at Massachusetts General Hospital, Boston, when Horace Wells, his former dental partner, attempted unsuccessfully to demonstrate the anodyne properties of nitrous oxide gas. Determined to find a more reliable pain-killing chemical, Morton consulted his former teacher, Boston chemist Charles Jackson, with whom he had previously done work on pain relief. The two discussed the use of ether, and Morton first used it in extraction of a tooth on Sept. 30, 1846. On October 16 he successfully demonstrated its use, administering ether to a patient undergoing a tumour operation in the same theatre where Wells had failed nearly two years earlier. A few weeks after Morton's demonstration, ether was used during a leg amputation performed by Robert Liston at University College Hospital in London.

Unfortunately, Morton attempted to obtain exclusive rights to the use of ether anesthesia. He spent the remainder of his life engaged in a costly contention with Jackson, who claimed priority in the discovery, despite official recognition accorded to Wells and the rural Georgia physician Crawford Long.

FLORENCE NIGHTINGALE
(born May 12, 1820, Florence [Italy]–died Aug. 13, 1910, London, England)

Florence Nightingale (byname Lady with the Lamp) was the foundational philosopher of modern nursing, a statistician, and a social reformer. Nightingale was put in charge of nursing British and allied soldiers in Turkey during the Crimean War. She spent many hours in the wards, and her night rounds giving personal care to the wounded established her image as the "Lady with the Lamp." Her efforts to formalize nursing education led her to establish the first scientifically based nursing school—the Nightingale School of Nursing, at St. Thomas' Hospital in London (opened 1860). She also was instrumental in setting up training for midwives and nurses in workhouse infirmaries. She was the first woman awarded the Order of Merit (1907). International Nurses Day, observed annually on May 12, commemorates her birth and celebrates the important role of nurses in health care.

Family Ties and Spiritual Awakening

Florence Nightingale was the second of two daughters born, during an extended European honeymoon, to William Edward and Frances Nightingale. (William Edward's original surname was Shore; he changed his name to Nightingale after inheriting his great-uncle's estate in 1815.) Florence was named after the city of her birth. After returning to England in 1821, the Nightingales had a comfortable lifestyle, dividing their time between two homes, Lea Hurst in Derbyshire, located in central

England, and Embley Park in warmer Hampshire, located in south-central England. Embley Park, a large and comfortable estate, became the primary family residence, with the Nightingales taking trips to Lea Hurst in the summer and to London during the social season.

Florence was a precocious child intellectually. Her father took particular interest in her education, guiding her through history, philosophy, and literature. She excelled in mathematics and languages and was able to read and write French, German, Italian, Greek, and Latin at an early age. Never satisfied with the traditional female skills of home management, she preferred to read the great philosophers and to engage in serious political and social discourse with her father.

As part of a liberal Unitarian family, Florence found great comfort in her religious beliefs. At the age of 16, she experienced one of several "calls from God." She viewed her particular calling as reducing human suffering. Nursing seemed the suitable route to serve both God and humankind. However, despite having cared for sick relatives and tenants on the family estates, her attempts to seek nurse's training were thwarted by her family as an inappropriate activity for a woman of her stature.

Nursing in Peace and War

Despite family reservations, Nightingale was eventually able to enroll at the Institution of Protestant Deaconesses at Kaiserswerth in Germany for two weeks of training in July 1850 and again for three months in July 1851. There she learned basic nursing skills, the importance of patient observation, and the value of good hospital organization. In 1853 Nightingale sought to break free from her family environment. Through social connections, she became the superintendent of the Institution for Sick Gentlewomen (governesses) in Distressed Circumstances, in London, where she successfully displayed her skills as an administrator by improving nursing care, working conditions, and efficiency of the hospital. After one year she began to realize that her services would be more valuable in an institution that would allow her to train nurses. She considered becoming the superintendent of nurses at King's College Hospital in London. However, politics, not nursing expertise, was to shape her next move.

In October 1853 the Turkish Ottoman Empire declared war on Russia, following a series of disputes over holy places in Jerusalem and Russian demands to exercise protection over the Orthodox subjects of the Ottoman sultan. The British and the French, allies of Turkey, sought to curb Russian expansion. The majority of the Crimean War was fought on the Crimean Peninsula in Russia. However, the British troop base and hospitals for the care of the sick and wounded soldiers were primarily established in Scutari (Üsküdar), across the Bosporus from Constantinople (Istanbul). The status of the care of the wounded was reported to the London *Times* by the first modern war correspondent, British journalist William Howard Russell. The newspaper reports stated that soldiers were treated by an incompetent and ineffective medical establishment and that the most basic supplies were not available for care. The British public raised an outcry over the treatment of the soldiers and demanded that the situation be drastically improved.

Sidney Herbert, secretary of state at war for the British government, wrote to Nightingale requesting that she lead a group of nurses to Scutari. At the same time, Nightingale wrote to her friend Liz Herbert, Sidney's wife, asking that she be allowed to lead a private expedition. Their letters crossed in the mail, but in the end their mutual requests were granted. Nightingale led an officially sanctioned party of 38 women, departing Oct. 21, 1854, and arriving in Scutari at the Barrack Hospital on November 5. Not welcomed by the medical officers, Nightingale found conditions filthy, supplies inadequate, staff uncooperative, and overcrowding severe. Few nurses had access to the cholera wards, and Nightingale, who wanted to gain the confidence of army surgeons by waiting for official military orders for assistance, kept her party from the wards. Five days after Nightingale's arrival in Scutari, injured soldiers from the Battle of Balaklava and the Battle of Inkerman arrived and overwhelmed the facility. Nightingale said it was the "Kingdom of Hell."

In order to care for the soldiers properly, it was necessary that adequate supplies be obtained. Nightingale bought equipment with funds provided by the London *Times* and enlisted soldiers' wives to assist with the laundry. The wards were cleaned and basic care was provided by the nurses. Most important, Nightingale established standards of care, requiring such basic necessities as bathing, clean clothing and dressings, and adequate food. Attention was given to

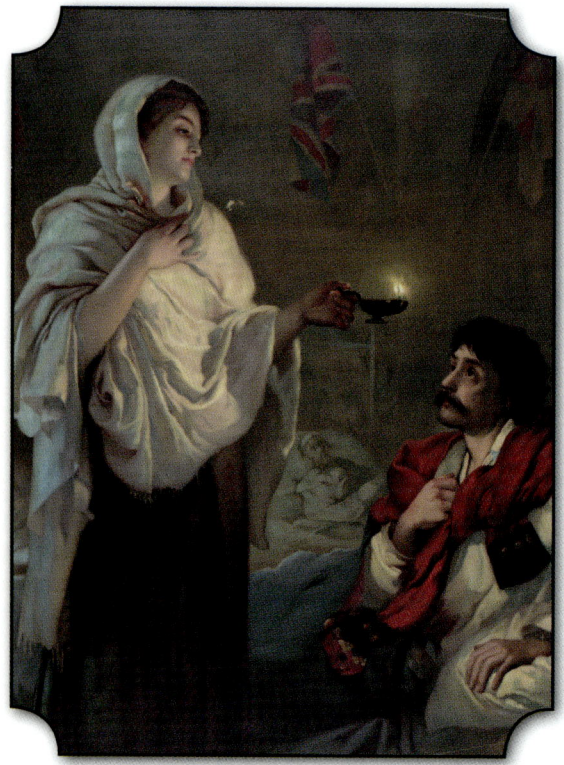

Florence Nightingale, with her signature lamp, visits patients during the Crimean War.

psychological needs through assistance in writing letters to relatives and through providing educational and recreational activities. Nightingale herself wandered the wards at night, providing support to the patients; this earned her the title of "Lady with the Lamp." She gained the respect of the soldiers and medical establishment alike. Her accomplishments in providing care and reportedly reducing the mortality rate to about 2 percent brought her fame in England through the press and the soldiers' letters. (Investigations by historians in the 20th century revealed that the mortality rate at Barrack Hospital under Nightingale's care was actually much higher than had been reported—the British government had concealed the actual mortality rate.)

In May 1855 Nightingale began the first of several excursions to Crimea; however, shortly after arriving, she fell ill with "Crimean fever"—most likely brucellosis, which she probably contracted from drinking contaminated milk. Nightingale experienced a slow recovery, as no active treatment was available. The lingering effects of the disease were to last for 25 years, frequently confining her to bed because of severe chronic pain.

On March 30, 1856, the Treaty of Paris ended the Crimean War. Nightingale remained in Scutari until the hospitals were ready to close, returning to her home in Derbyshire on Aug. 7, 1856, as a reluctant heroine.

Homecoming and Legacy

Although primarily remembered for her accomplishments during the Crimean War, Nightingale's greatest achievements centred on attempts to create social reform in health care and nursing. On her return to England, Nightingale was suffering the effects of both brucellosis and exhaustion. In September 1856 she met with Queen

Victoria and Prince Albert to discuss the need for reform of the British military establishment. Nightingale kept meticulous records regarding the running of the Barrack Hospital, causes of illness and death, the efficiency of the nursing and medical staffs, and difficulties in purveyance. A Royal Commission was established, which based its findings on the statistical data and analysis provided by Nightingale. The result was marked reform in the military medical and purveyance systems.

In 1855, as a token of gratitude and respect for Nightingale, the Nightingale Fund was established. Through private donations, £45,000 was raised by 1859 and put at Nightingale's disposal. She used a substantial part of these monies to institute the Nightingale School of Nursing at St. Thomas' Hospital in London, which opened in 1860. The school formalized secular nursing education, making nursing a viable and respectable option for women who desired employment outside of the home. The model was taken worldwide by matrons (women supervisors of public health institutions). Nightingale's statistical models—such as the Coxcomb chart, which she developed to assess mortality—and her basic concepts regarding nursing remain applicable today. For these reasons she is considered the foundational philosopher of modern nursing.

Nightingale improved the health of households through her most famous publication, *Notes on Nursing: What It Is and What It Is Not*, which provided direction on how to manage the sick. This volume has been in continuous publication worldwide since 1859. Additional reforms were financed through the Nightingale Fund, and a school for the education of midwives was established at King's College Hospital in 1862. Believing that the most important location for the care of the sick was in the home, she established training for district nursing, which was aimed at improving the health of the poor and vulnerable. A second Royal Commission examined the health of India, resulting in major environmental reform, again based on Nightingale's statistical data.

Florence Nightingale was honoured in her lifetime by receiving the title of Lady of Grace of the Order of St. John of Jerusalem and by becoming the first woman to receive the Order of Merit. On her death in 1910, at Nightingale's prior request, her family declined the offer of a state funeral and burial in Westminster Abbey. Instead, she was honoured with a memorial service at St. Paul's Cathedral, London. Her burial is in the family plot in St. Margaret's Church, East Wellow, Hampshire.

ELIZABETH BLACKWELL
(born Feb. 3, 1821, Counterslip, Bristol, Gloucestershire, England–died May 31, 1910, Hastings, Sussex)

Elizabeth Blackwell was an Anglo-American physician who is considered the first woman doctor of medicine in modern times. Blackwell was from a large, prosperous, and cultured family and was well educated by private tutors. Financial reverses and the family's liberal social and religious views prompted them to immigrate to the United States in the summer of 1832. Soon after taking up residence in New York, her father, Samuel Blackwell, became active in abolitionist activities. The Blackwells moved to Jersey City, N.J., in 1835 and to Cincinnati, Ohio, in 1838. Soon afterward Samuel Blackwell's death left the family in poverty, and Elizabeth and two sisters opened a private school. Later Elizabeth taught school in Henderson, Ky,. and in 1845–47 in North and South Carolina.

During the latter period Elizabeth Blackwell undertook the study of medicine privately with sympathetic physicians, and in 1847 she began seeking admission to a medical school. All the leading schools rejected her application, but she was at length admitted, almost by fluke, to Geneva Medical College (a forerunner of Hobart College) in Geneva, New York. Her months there were extremely difficult. Townspeople and much of the male student body ostracized and harassed her, and she was at first even barred from classroom demonstration. She persevered, however, and in January 1849, ranked first in her class, she became the first woman in the United States to graduate from medical school and the first modern-day woman doctor of medicine.

In April, having become a naturalized U.S. citizen, Blackwell traveled to England to seek further training, and in May she went on to Paris, where in June she entered the midwives' course at La Maternité. While there she contracted an infectious eye disease that left her blind in one eye and forced her to abandon hope of becoming a surgeon. In October 1850 she returned to England and worked at St. Bartholomew's Hospital under Dr. (later Sir) James Paget. In the summer of 1851 she returned to New York, where she was refused posts in the city's hospitals and dispensaries and was even unable to rent private consulting quarters. Her private practice was very slow to develop, and in the meantime she wrote a series of lectures, published in 1852 as *The Laws of Life, with Special Reference to the Physical Education of Girls.*

In 1853 Blackwell opened a small dispensary in a slum district. Within a few years she was joined by her younger sister, Dr. Emily Blackwell, and by Dr. Marie E. Zakrzewska, and in May 1857 the dispensary, greatly enlarged, was incorporated as the New York Infirmary for Women and Children. In January 1859, during a year-long lecture tour of Great Britain, she became the first woman to have her name placed on the British medical register. At the outbreak of the American Civil War in 1861, she helped organize the Woman's Central Association of Relief and the U.S. Sanitary Commission and worked mainly through the former to select and train nurses for war service.

In November 1868 a plan long in the perfecting, developed in large part in consultation with Florence Nightingale in England, bore fruit in the opening of the Woman's Medical College at the infirmary. Elizabeth Blackwell set very high standards for admission, academic and clinical training, and certification for the school, which continued in operation for 31 years; she herself occupied the chair of hygiene. In 1869 Blackwell moved permanently to England. She established a successful private practice, helped organize the National Health Society in 1871, and in 1875 was appointed professor of gynecology at the London School of Medicine for Women. She retained the latter position until 1907, when an injury forced her to retire. Among her other writings are *The Religion of Health* (1871), *Counsel to Parents on the Moral Education of Their Children* (1878), *The Human Element in Sex* (1884), her autobiographical *Pioneer Work in Opening the Medical Profession to Women* (1895), and *Essays in Medical Sociology* (1902).

RUDOLF VIRCHOW

(born Oct. 13, 1821, Schivelbein, Pomerania, Prussia [now Swidwin, Poland]–died Sept. 5, 1902, Berlin, Germany)

Rudolf Virchow (in full Rudolf Carl Virchow) was a German pathologist and statesman, one of the most prominent physicians of the 19th century. He pioneered the modern concept of pathological processes by his application of the cell theory to explain the effects of disease in the organs and tissues of the body. He emphasized that diseases arose, not in organs or tissues in general, but primarily in their individual cells. Moreover, he campaigned vigorously for social reforms and contributed to the development of anthropology as a modern science.

Early Career

In 1839 Virchow began the study of medicine at the Friedrich Wilhelm Institute of the University of Berlin and was graduated as a doctor of medicine in 1843. As an intern at the Charité Hospital, he studied pathological histology and in 1845 published a paper in which he described one of the two earliest reported cases of leukemia. This paper became a classic. Virchow was appointed prosector at the Charité, and in 1847 he began, with his friend Benno Reinhardt, a new journal, *Archiv für pathologische Anatomie und Physiologie, und für klinische Medizin* (*Archives for Pathological Anatomy and Physiology, and for Clinical Medicine*). After Reinhardt's death in 1852, Virchow continued as sole editor of the journal, later known as *Virchows Archiv*, until his own death 50 years later.

Early in 1848 Virchow was appointed by the Prussian government to investigate an outbreak of typhus in Upper Silesia; his subsequent report laid the blame for the outbreak on social conditions and on the government. The government was annoyed, but it had to deal with the revolution of 1848 in Berlin. Eight days after his return from Silesia, Virchow was fighting at the barricades. After the revolution Virchow embraced the cause of such medical reforms as abolition of the various grades of physicians and surgeons, and from July 1848 to June 1849 he published a weekly paper, *Die Medizinische Reform* (*Medical Reform*) much of which he wrote himself. His liberal views led the government, on March 31, 1849, to suspend him from his post at the Charité, but a fortnight later he was reinstated, with the loss of certain privileges.

Later in 1849, Virchow was appointed to the newly established chair of pathological anatomy at the University of Würzburg—the first chair of that subject in Germany. During his seven fruitful years in that post, the number of medical students in the university increased from 98 to 388. Many men who later attained fame in the medical field received training there from him. In 1850 he married Rose Mayer, with whom he had three sons and three daughters. At Würzburg Virchow published many papers on pathological anatomy. He began there the publication of his six-volume *Handbuch der speziellen Pathologie und Therapie* (*Handbook of Special Pathology and Therapeutics*), most of the first volume of which he wrote himself. At Würzburg he also began to formulate his theories on cellular pathology and started his anthropological work with studies of the abnormal skulls of individuals affected by cretinism (a condition later recognized as neonatal hypothyroidism) and investigations into the development of the base of the skull.

In 1856 a chair of pathological anatomy was established for Virchow at the University of Berlin; he accepted the call subject to certain conditions, one of which was the erection of a new pathological institute, which he used for the rest of his life. During much of this second Berlin period, Virchow actively engaged in politics. In 1859 he was elected to the Berlin City Council, focusing his attention on public health matters, such as sewage disposal, the design of hospitals, meat inspection, and school hygiene. He supervised the design of two large new Berlin hospitals, the Friedrichshain and the Moabit, opened a nursing school in the Friedrichshain Hospital, and designed the new Berlin sewer system.

In 1861 Virchow was elected to the Prussian Diet. He

was a founder of the Fortschrittspartei (Progressive Party) and a determined and untiring opponent of Otto von Bismarck, who in 1865 challenged him to a duel, which he wisely declined. In the wars of 1866 and 1870 Virchow confined his political activities to the erection of military hospitals and the equipping of hospital trains. In the Franco-German War he personally led the first hospital train to the front. He was a member of the Reichstag from 1880 to 1893.

Medical Investigations

By 1848 Virchow had disproved a prominent view that phlebitis (inflammation of a vein) causes most diseases. He demonstrated that masses in the blood vessels resulted from "thrombosis" (his term, meaning the formation or presence of a blood clot in a blood vessel) and that portions of a thrombus could become detached to form an "embolus" (also his term, meaning a clot that has broken free from its point of origin). An embolus set free in the circulation might eventually be trapped in a narrower vessel and lead to a serious lesion in the neighbouring parts.

Virchow's concept of cellular pathology was initiated while he was at Würzburg. Until the latter part of the 18th century, diseases were supposed to be due to an imbalance of the four fluid humours of the body (blood, phlegm, yellow bile, and black bile). This was the "humoural pathology," which dated back to the Greeks. In 1761 an Italian anatomist, Giovanni Battista Morgagni, showed that diseases were due not to an imbalance of the humours but to lesions in organs. Around 1800 French anatomist Marie-François-Xavier Bichat demonstrated that the body was made up of 21 different kinds of tissues, and he conceived that in a diseased organ only some of its tissues might be affected. The later events in the complex history of the cell theory were taking place while Virchow was a youth. Recognizing that the basic problem was the origin of cells, early investigators invented a hypothesis of "free cell formation," according to which cells developed *de novo* out of an unformed substance, a "cytoblastema," by a sequence of events in which first the nucleolus develops, followed by the nucleus, the cell body, and finally the cell membrane. The best physical model of the generation of formed bodies then available was crystallization, and their theory was inspired by that model. In retrospect, the hypothesis of free cell formation would not seem to have been justified, however, since cell division, a feature not characteristic of crystallization processes, had frequently been observed by earlier microscopists, especially among single-celled organisms. Even though cell division was observed repeatedly in the following decades, the theory of free cell formation lingered throughout most of the 19th century; however, it came to be thought of more and more as a possible exception to the general principle of the reproduction of cells by division.

At Würzburg Virchow began to realize that one form of the cell theory, which postulated that every cell originated from a preexisting cell rather than from amorphous material, could give new insight into pathological processes. In this he was influenced by the work of many others, notably by the views of John Goodsir of Edinburgh on the cell as a centre of nutrition and by the investigations of Robert Remak, a German neuroanatomist and embryologist, who in 1852 was one of the first to point out that cell division accounted for the multiplication of cells to form tissues. By that year Remak had concluded that new cells arose from existing cells in diseased as well as healthy tissue. Remak's writings, however, had little influence on pathologists and medical practitioners. Thus the idea expressed by Virchow's *omnis cellula e cellula* ("every cell is derived from a [preexisting] cell") is not completely original. Even this aphorism is not Virchow's; it was coined by François Vincent Raspail in 1825. But Virchow made cellular pathology into a system of overwhelming importance. His main statement of the theory was given in a series of 20 lectures in 1858. The lectures, published in 1858 as his book *Die Cellularpathologie in ihrer Begründung auf physiologische und pathologische Gewebenlehre* (*Cellular Pathology as Based upon Physiological and Pathological Histology*), at once transformed scientific thought in the whole field of biology.

Virchow shed new light on the process of inflammation, though he erroneously rejected the possibility of migration of the leukocytes (white blood cells). He distinguished between fatty infiltration (an abnormal depositing of fat globules on tissue) and fatty degeneration (an abnormal depositing of fat globules, which causes tissue to deteriorate), and he introduced the modern conception of amyloid (starchy) degeneration. He devoted great attention to the pathology of tumours, but the importance of his papers on malignant tumours and of his three-volume work on that subject (*Die krankhaften Geschwülste,* 1863–67) was somewhat marred by his erroneous conception that malignancy results from a conversion (metaplasia) of connective tissue. His work on the role of animal parasites, especially trichina, in causing disease in humans was fundamental and led to his own public interest in meat inspection. In 1874 he introduced a standardized technique for performing autopsies, by the use of which the whole body was examined in detail, often revealing unsuspected lesions.

Virchow's attitude to the new science of bacteriology was complex. He was somewhat resistant to the idea that bacteria had a role in causing disease, and he rightly argued that the presence of a certain microorganism in a patient with a particular disease did not always indicate that that organism was the cause of the disease. He suggested, long before toxins were actually discovered, that some bacteria might produce these substances. Though it is sometimes said that Virchow was antagonistic to Charles Darwin's theory of the origin of species by natural selection, the fact is that he accepted the theory as a hypothesis but maintained throughout his later years that there was insufficient scientific evidence to justify its full acceptance.

Work in Anthropology

In 1865 Virchow discovered pile dwellings in northern Germany, and in 1870 he started to excavate hill forts. Meanwhile he had been using his enormous influence in the cause of anthropology. In 1869 he was part founder of the German Anthropological Society, and in the same year he founded the Berlin Society for Anthropology, Ethnology, and Prehistory, of which he was president from 1869 until his death. During the whole of that period, he edited its *Zeitschrift für Ethnologie* (*Journal of Ethnology*).

In 1874 Virchow met Heinrich Schliemann, the discoverer of the site of Troy, and he accompanied Schliemann to Troy in 1879 and to Egypt in 1888. It was due largely to Virchow that Schliemann gave his magnificent collection to Berlin. In 1881 and in 1894 Virchow made personal expeditions to the Caucasus. Virchow was the organizer of German anthropology.

In 1873 Virchow was elected to the Prussian Academy of Sciences. He declined to be ennobled as "von Virchow," but in 1894 he was created *Geheimrat* ("privy councillor").

CLARA BARTON

(born Dec. 25, 1821, Oxford, Mass., U.S.–died April 12, 1912, Glen Echo, Md.)

Clara Barton (in full Clarissa Harlowe Barton) was the founder of the American Red Cross. Barton was educated at home and began teaching at age 15. She attended the Liberal Institute at Clinton, N.Y. (1850–51). In 1852 in Bordentown, N.J., she established a free school that soon became so large that the townsmen would no longer allow a woman to run it. Rather than subordinate herself to a male principal, Barton resigned. She was then employed by the U.S. Patent Office in Washington, D.C., from 1854 to 1857 and again in 1860.

At the outbreak of the American Civil War, Barton showed characteristic initiative in organizing facilities to recover soldiers' lost baggage and in securing medicine and supplies for men wounded in the First Battle of Bull Run. She gained permission to pass through the battle lines to distribute supplies, search for the missing, and nurse the wounded. Barton carried on this work through the remainder of the Civil War, traveling with the army as far south as Charleston, S.C., in 1863. In June 1864 she was formally appointed superintendent of nurses for the Army of the James. In 1865, at the request of Pres. Abraham Lincoln, she set up a bureau of records to aid in the search for missing men.

While she was in Europe for a rest (1869–70), the Franco-German War broke out, and Barton again distributed relief supplies to war victims. In Europe she became associated with the International Red Cross (now Red Cross and Red Crescent), and after her return to the United States in 1873 she campaigned vigorously and successfully for that country to sign the Geneva Convention.

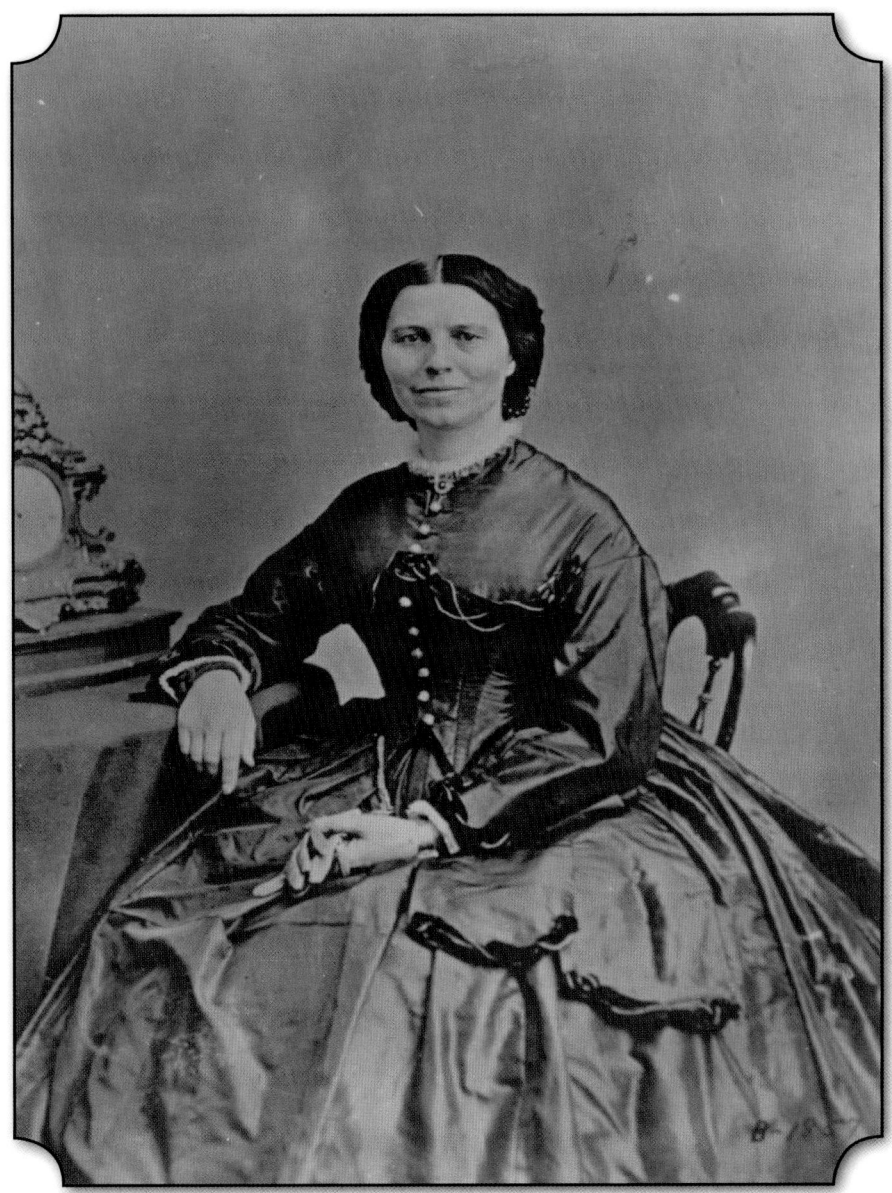

In addition to her contributions to nursing in the United States, Clara Barton organized the American National Red Cross.

The agreement sought to allow for the treating of the sick and wounded in battle, the proper identifying and burial of those killed in battle, and the proper handling of prisoners of war. In 1881 she organized the American Association of the Red Cross, known from 1893 as the American National Red Cross, and served as its president until 1904. She wrote the American amendment to the constitution of the Red Cross, which provides for the distribution of relief not only in war but also in times of such calamities as famines, floods, earthquakes, tornadoes, and pestilence.

Barton devoted herself entirely to the organization, soliciting contributions and taking to the field with relief workers even as late as the Spanish-American War in Cuba, when she was 77 years old. She was jealous of any interference, however, and supervised the organization's activities so closely that charges of authoritarianism were brought against her by members of the executive council. The Red Cross had been chartered by Congress in 1900, and the rebelling faction used that lever to force Barton's resignation in 1904. Despite the arbitrariness of her administrative methods, her achievements remained; she was affectionately known as the "angel of the battlefield" for her life's work. She wrote several books, including *History of the Red Cross* (1882), *The Red Cross in Peace and War* (1899), and *The Story of My Childhood* (1907).

Through its affiliation with the International Red Cross and Red Crescent, the American Red Cross continues to travel internationally to provide disaster relief and establish development programs. In addition to providing disaster relief, the American Red Cross oversees the collection, testing, storage, and distribution of blood donations. Other services include community assistance to the economically disadvantaged, support for members of the military and their families, and health and safety education, such as cardiopulmonary resuscitation (CPR), first aid, and lifeguarding classes. As with any other public health service organization, advocacy is part of the essential work of the American Red Cross in its mission to serve and protect the public. Therefore, it works with legislators and administrators at all levels of government to pursue the public interest. The advocacy function involves developing policy statements, testifying at hearings, generating position statements, and serving on external task forces and committees.

LOUIS PASTEUR

(born Dec. 27, 1822, Dole, France–died Sept. 28, 1895, Saint-Cloud)

Louis Pasteur was a French chemist and microbiologist who was one of the most important founders of medical microbiology. Pasteur's contributions to science, technology, and medicine are nearly without precedent. He pioneered the study of molecular asymmetry; discovered that microorganisms cause fermentation and disease; originated the process of pasteurization; saved the beer, wine, and silk industries in France; and developed vaccines against anthrax and rabies.

Pasteur's academic positions were numerous, and his scientific accomplishments earned him France's highest decoration, the Legion of Honour, as well as election to the Académie des Sciences and many other distinctions. Today there are some 30 institutes and an impressive number of hospitals, schools, buildings, and streets that bear his name—a set of honours bestowed on few scientists.

Early Education

Pasteur's father, Jean-Joseph Pasteur, was a tanner and a sergeant major decorated with the Legion of Honour during the Napoleonic Wars. This fact probably instilled in the younger Pasteur the strong patriotism that later was a defining element of his character. Louis Pasteur was an average student in his early years, but he was gifted in drawing and painting. His pastels and portraits of his parents and friends, made when he was 15, were later kept in the museum of the Pasteur Institute in Paris. After attending primary school in Arbois, where his family had moved, and secondary school in nearby Besançon, he earned his bachelor of arts degree (1840) and bachelor of science degree (1842) at the Royal College of Besançon.

Research Career

In 1843 Pasteur was admitted to the École Normale Supérieure (a teachers' college in Paris), where he attended lectures by French chemist Jean-Baptiste-André Dumas and became Dumas's teaching assistant. Pasteur obtained his master of science degree in 1845 and then acquired an advanced degree in physical sciences. He later earned his doctorate in sciences in 1847. Pasteur was appointed professor of physics at the Dijon Lycée (secondary school) in 1848 but shortly thereafter accepted a position as professor of chemistry at the University of Strasbourg. On May 29, 1849, he married Marie Laurent, the daughter of the rector of the university. The couple had five children; however, only two survived childhood.

Molecular Asymmetry

Soon after graduating from the École Normale Supérieure, Pasteur became puzzled by the discovery of the German chemist Eilhardt Mitscherlich, who had shown that tartrates and paratartrates (both salts of soda and ammonia) behaved differently toward polarized light (optical activity is the ability of a substance to rotate the plane of polarization of a beam of light that is passed through it): tartrates rotated the plane of polarized light, whereas paratartrates did not. This was unusual because the compounds displayed identical chemical properties.

In physics, symmetry is the concept that the properties of particles such as atoms and molecules remain unchanged after being subjected to a variety of symmetry transformations or "operations." Valid symmetry operations are those that can be performed without changing the appearance of an object. Pasteur noted that the tartrate crystals exhibited asymmetric forms that corresponded to their optical asymmetry. He made the surprising observation that crystalline paratartrate consisted of a mixture of crystals in a right-handed configuration. However, when these crystals were separated manually, he found that they exhibited right and left asymmetry. In other words, a balanced mixture of both right and left crystals was optically inactive. Thus, Pasteur discovered the existence of molecular asymmetry, the foundation of stereochemistry, as it was revealed by optical activity. Over the course of the next 10 years, Pasteur further investigated the ability of organic substances to rotate the plane of polarized light. He also studied the relationship that existed between crystal structure and molecular configuration. His studies convinced him that asymmetry was one of the fundamental characteristics of living matter.

Germ Theory of Fermentation

In 1854 Pasteur was appointed professor of chemistry and dean of the science faculty at the University of Lille. While working at Lille, he was asked to help solve problems related to alcohol production at a local distillery, and thus he began a series of studies on alcoholic fermentation (the chemical process by which molecules such as glucose are broken down anaerobically). His work on these problems led to his involvement in tackling a variety of other practical and economic problems involving fermentation. His efforts proved successful in unraveling most of these problems, and new theoretical implications emerged from his work. Pasteur investigated a broad range of aspects of fermentation, including the production of compounds such as lactic acid that are responsible for the souring of milk. He also studied butyric acid fermentation.

In 1857 Pasteur left Lille and returned to Paris, having been appointed manager and director of scientific studies at the École Normale Supérieure. That same year he presented experimental evidence for the participation of living organisms in all fermentative processes and showed that a specific organism was associated with each particular fermentation. This evidence gave rise to the germ theory of fermentation.

Pasteur Effect

The realization that specific organisms were involved in fermentation was further supported by Pasteur's studies of butyric acid fermentation. These studies led Pasteur to the unexpected discovery that the fermentation process could be arrested by passing air (that is, oxygen) through the fermenting fluid, a process known today as the Pasteur effect. He concluded that this was due to the presence of a life-form that could function only in the absence of oxygen. This led to his introduction of the terms *aerobic* and *anaerobic* to designate organisms that live in the presence or absence of oxygen, respectively. He further proposed that the phenomena occurring during putrefaction were due to specific germs that function under anaerobic conditions.

Pasteurization

Pasteur readily applied his knowledge of microbes and fermentation to the wine and beer industries in France, effectively saving the industries from collapse due to problems associated with production and with contamination that occurred during export. In 1863, at the request of the emperor of France, Napoleon III, Pasteur studied wine contamination and showed it to be caused by microbes. To prevent contamination, Pasteur used a simple procedure: he heated the wine to 50–60 °C (120–140 °F), a process now known universally as pasteurization. Today pasteurization is seldom used for wines that benefit from aging, since it kills the organisms that contribute to the aging process, but it is applied to many foods and beverages, particularly milk.

Following Pasteur's success with wine, he focused his studies on beer. By developing practical techniques for the control of beer fermentation, he was able to provide a rational methodology for the brewing industry. He also devised a method for the manufacturing of beer that prevented deterioration of the product during long periods of transport on ships.

Spontaneous Generation

Fermentation and putrefaction were often perceived as being spontaneous phenomena, a perception stemming from the ancient belief that life could generate spontaneously. During the 18th century the debate was pursued by the English naturalist and Roman Catholic divine John Turberville Needham and the French naturalist Georges-Louis Leclerc, count de Buffon. While both supported the idea of spontaneous generation, Italian abbot and physiologist Lazzaro Spallanzani maintained that life could never spontaneously generate from dead matter. In 1859, the year English naturalist Charles Darwin published his *On the Origin of Species*, Pasteur decided to settle this dispute. He was convinced that his germ theory could not be firmly substantiated as long as belief in spontaneous generation persisted. Pasteur attacked the problem by using a simple experimental procedure. He showed that beef broth could be sterilized by boiling it in a "swan-neck" flask, which has a long bending neck that traps dust particles and other contaminants before they reach the body of the flask. However, if the broth was boiled and the neck of the flask was broken off following boiling, the broth, being reexposed to air, eventually became cloudy, indicating microbial contamination. These experiments proved that there was no spontaneous generation, since the boiled broth, if never reexposed to air, remained sterile. This not only settled the philosophical problem of the origin of life at the time but also placed on solid ground the new science of bacteriology, which relied on proven techniques of sterilization and aseptic manipulation.

Work with Silkworms

In 1862 Pasteur was elected to the Académie des Sciences, and the following year he was appointed professor of geology, physics, and chemistry at the École des Beaux-Arts (School of Fine Arts). Shortly after this, Pasteur turned his attention to France's silkworm crisis. In the middle of the 19th century, a mysterious disease had attacked French silkworm nurseries. Silkworm eggs could no longer be produced in France, and they could not be imported from other countries, since the disease had spread all over Europe and had invaded the Caucasus region of Eurasia, as well as China and Japan. By 1865 the silkworm industry

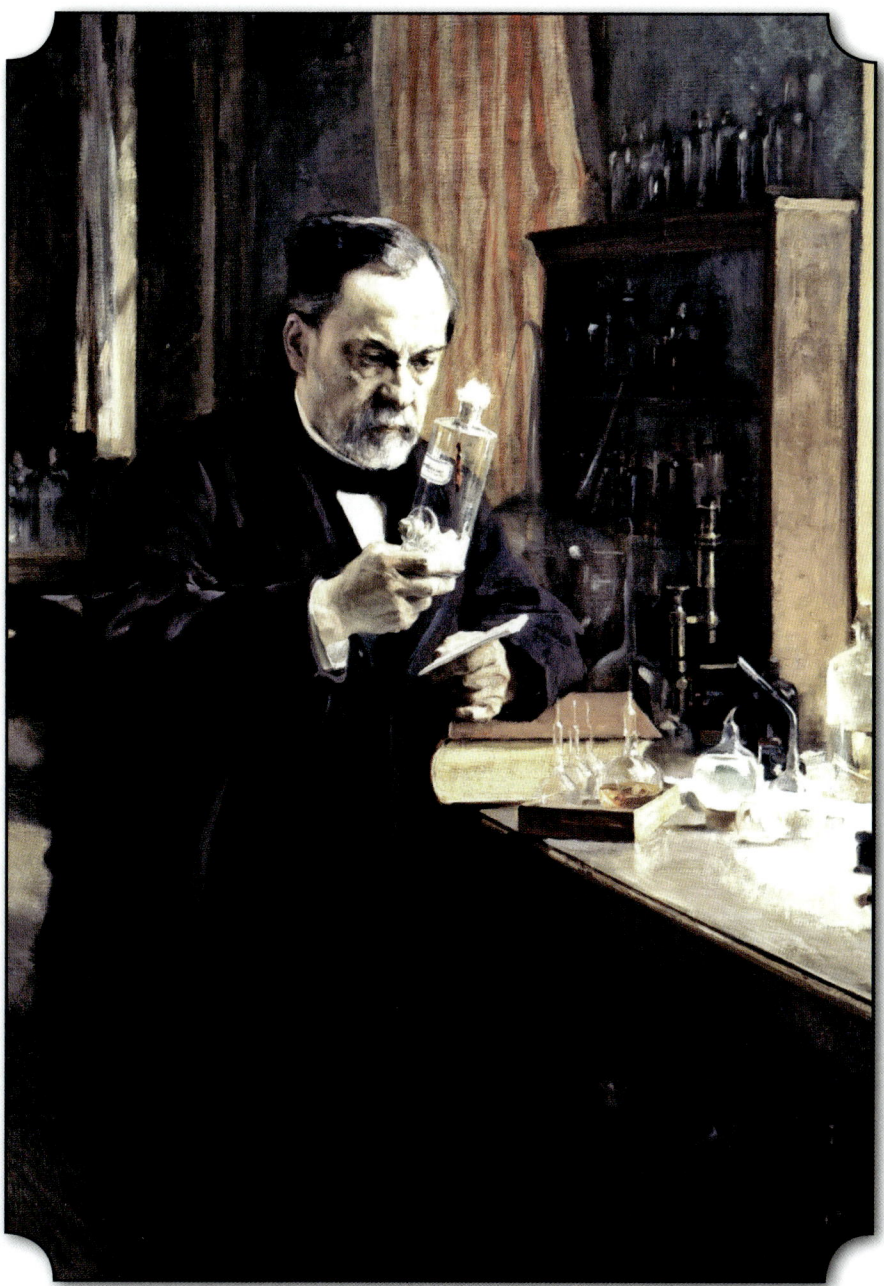

This 1885 painting by Albert Edelfelt depicts Louis Pasteur in his laboratory.

was almost completely ruined in France and, to a lesser extent, in the rest of western Europe. Pasteur knew virtually nothing about silkworms, but, upon the request of his former mentor Dumas, Pasteur took charge of the problem, accepting the challenge and seizing the opportunity to learn more about infectious diseases. He soon became an expert silkworm breeder and identified the organisms that caused the silkworm disease. After five years of research, he succeeded in saving the silk industry through a method that enabled the preservation of healthy silkworm eggs and prevented their contamination by the disease-causing organisms. Within a couple of years, this method was recognized throughout Europe; it is still used today in silk-producing countries.

In 1867 Pasteur resigned from his administrative duties at the École Normale Supérieure and was appointed professor of chemistry at the Sorbonne, a university in Paris. Although he was partially paralyzed (left hemiplegia) in 1868, he continued his research. For Pasteur, the study of silkworms constituted an initiation into the problem of infectious diseases, and it was then that he first became aware of the complexities of infectious processes. Accustomed as he was to the constancy and accuracy of laboratory procedures, he was puzzled by the variability of animal life, which he had come to recognize through his observation that individual silkworms differed in their response to disease depending on physiological and environmental factors. By investigating these problems, Pasteur developed certain practices of epidemiology that served him well a few years later when he dealt with animal and human diseases.

Vaccine Development

In the early 1870s Pasteur had already acquired considerable renown and respect in France, and in 1873 he was elected as an associate member of the Académie de Médecine. Nonetheless, the medical establishment was reluctant to accept his germ theory of disease, primarily because it originated from a chemist. However, during the next decade, Pasteur developed the overall principle of vaccination and contributed to the foundation of immunology.

Pasteur's first important discovery in the study of vaccination came in 1879 and concerned a disease called chicken cholera. (Today the bacteria that cause the disease are classified in the genus *Pasteurella*.) Pasteur said, "Chance only favours the prepared mind," and it was chance observation through which he discovered that cultures of chicken cholera lost their pathogenicity (ability to cause disease) and retained "attenuated" pathogenic characteristics over the course of many generations. He inoculated chickens with the attenuated form and demonstrated that the chickens were resistant to the fully virulent strain. From then on, Pasteur directed all his experimental work toward the problem of immunization and applied this principle to many other diseases.

Pasteur began investigating anthrax in 1879. At that time an anthrax epidemic in France and in some other parts of Europe had killed a large number of sheep, and the disease was attacking humans as well. German physician Robert Koch announced the isolation of the anthrax bacillus, which Pasteur confirmed. Koch and Pasteur independently provided definitive experimental evidence that the anthrax bacillus was indeed responsible for the infection. This firmly established the germ theory of disease, which then emerged as the fundamental concept underlying medical microbiology.

Pasteur wanted to apply the principle of vaccination to anthrax. He prepared attenuated cultures of the bacillus after determining the conditions that led to the organism's loss of virulence. In the spring of 1881 he obtained financial support, mostly from farmers, to conduct a large-scale public experiment of anthrax immunization. The experiment took place in Pouilly-le-Fort, located on the southern outskirts of Paris. Pasteur immunized 70 farm animals, and the experiment was a complete success. The vaccination procedure involved two inoculations at intervals of 12 days with vaccines of different potencies. One vaccine, from a low-virulence culture, was given to half the sheep and was followed by a second vaccine from a more virulent culture than the first. Two weeks after these initial inoculations, both the vaccinated and control sheep were inoculated with a virulent strain of anthrax. Within a few days all the control sheep died, whereas all the vaccinated animals survived. This convinced many people that Pasteur's work was indeed valid.

Following the success of the anthrax vaccination experiment, Pasteur focused on the microbial origins of disease. His investigations of animals infected by pathogenic microbes and his studies of the microbial mechanisms that cause harmful physiological effects in animals made him a pioneer in the field of infectious pathology. It is often said that English surgeon Edward Jenner discovered vaccination and that Pasteur invented vaccines. Indeed, almost 90 years after Jenner initiated immunization against smallpox, Pasteur developed another vaccine—the first vaccine against rabies. He had decided to attack the problem of rabies in 1882, the year of his acceptance into the Académie Française. Rabies was a dreaded and horrible disease that had fascinated popular imagination for centuries because of its mysterious origin and the fear it generated. Conquering it would be Pasteur's final endeavour.

Pasteur suspected that the agent that caused rabies

was a microbe (the agent was later discovered to be a virus, a nonliving entity). It was too small to be seen under Pasteur's microscope, and so experimentation with the disease demanded the development of entirely new methodologies. Pasteur chose to conduct his experiments using rabbits and transmitted the infectious agent from animal to animal by intracerebral inoculations until he obtained a stable preparation. In order to attenuate the invisible agent, he desiccated the spinal cords of infected animals until the preparation became almost nonvirulent. He realized later that, instead of creating an attenuated form of the agent, his treatment had actually neutralized it. (Pasteur perceived the neutralizing effect as a killing effect on the agent, since he suspected that the agent was a living organism.) Thus, rather unknowingly, he had produced, instead of attenuated live microorganisms, a neutralized agent and opened the way for the development of a second class of vaccines, known as inactivated vaccines.

On July 6, 1885, Pasteur vaccinated Joseph Meister, a nine-year-old boy who had been bitten by a rabid dog. The vaccine was so successful that it brought immediate glory and fame to Pasteur. Hundreds of other bite victims throughout the world were subsequently saved by Pasteur's vaccine, and the era of preventive medicine had begun. An international fund-raising campaign was launched to build the Pasteur Institute in Paris, the inauguration of which took place on Nov. 14, 1888.

IMPLICATIONS OF PASTEUR'S WORK

The theoretical implications and practical importance of Pasteur's work were immense. Pasteur once said, "There are no such things as pure and applied science; there are only science and the application of science." Thus, once he established the theoretical basis of a given process, he investigated ways to further develop industrial applications. (As a result, he deposited a number of patents.)

However, Pasteur did not have enough time to explore all the practical aspects of his numerous theories. One of the most important theoretical implications of his later research, which emerged from his attenuation procedure for vaccines, is the concept that virulence is not a constant attribute but a variable property—a property that can be lost and later recovered. Virulence could be decreased, but Pasteur suspected that it could be increased as well. He believed that increased virulence was what gave rise to epidemics. In *Louis Pasteur, Free Lance of Science* (1950), American microbiologist René Dubos quoted Pasteur:

> Thus, virulence appears in a new light which may be disturbing for the future of humanity unless nature, in its long evolution, has already had the occasions to produce all possible contagious diseases—a very unlikely assumption.
>
> What is a microorganism that is innocuous to man or to a given animal species? It is a living being which does not possess the capacity to multiply in our body or in the body of the animal. But nothing proves that if the same microorganism should chance to come into contact with some other of the thousands of animal species in the Creation, it might invade it and render it sick. Its virulence might increase by repeated passages through that species, and might eventually affect man or domesticated animals. Thus might be brought about a new virulence and new contagions. I am much inclined to believe that such mechanisms

would explain how smallpox, syphilis, plague, yellow fever, etc. have come about in the course of time, and how certain great epidemics appear once in a while.

Pasteur was the first to recognize variability in virulence. Today this concept remains relevant to the study of infectious disease, especially with regard to understanding the emergence of diseases such as bovine spongiform encephalopathy (BSE), severe acute respiratory syndrome (SARS), and acquired immunodeficiency syndrome (AIDS).

After Pasteur's 70th birthday, which was acknowledged by a large but solemn celebration at the Sorbonne that was attended by several prominent scientists, including British surgeon Joseph Lister, Pasteur's health continued to deteriorate. His paralysis worsened, and he died on Sept. 28, 1895. He was buried in the cathedral of Notre-Dame de Paris, but his remains were transferred to a Neo-Byzantine crypt at the Pasteur Institute in 1896.

During Pasteur's career, he touched on many problems, but a simple description of his achievements does not do justice to the intensity and fullness of his life. He never accepted defeat, and he always tried to convince skeptics, though his impatience and intolerance were notorious when he believed that truth was on his side. Throughout his life he was an immensely effective observer and readily integrated relevant observations into conceptual schemes.

JOSEPH LISTER, BARON LISTER OF LYME REGIS

(born April 5, 1827, Upton, Essex, England–died Feb. 10, 1912, Walmer, Kent)

Joseph Lister, (also called [1883–97] Sir Joseph Lister, Baronet) was a British surgeon and medical scientist who was the founder of antiseptic medicine and a pioneer in preventive medicine. While his method, based on the use of antiseptics, is no longer employed, his principle—that bacteria must never gain entry to an operation wound—remains the basis of surgery to this day. He was made a baronet in 1883 and raised to the peerage in 1897.

EDUCATION

Lister was the second son of Joseph Jackson Lister and his wife, Isabella Harris, members of the Society of Friends, or Quakers. J.J. Lister, a wine merchant and amateur physicist and microscopist, was elected a fellow of the Royal Society for his discovery that led to the modern achromatic (non-colour-distorting) microscope. He discovered a method of combining lenses that greatly improved image resolution by eliminating certain chromatic and spherical aberrations. In 1830 he began grinding his own lenses, developing techniques that he taught to optical instrument makers in London. Using his newly developed lenses, Lister was the first to determine the true form of the red blood cell in mammalian blood.

While both parents took an active part in Lister's education, his father instructing him in natural history and the use of the microscope, Lister received his formal schooling in two Quaker institutions, which laid far more emphasis upon natural history and science than did other schools. He became interested in comparative anatomy, and, before his 16th birthday, he had decided upon a surgical career.

After taking an arts course at University College, London, he enrolled in the faculty of medical science in October 1848. A brilliant student, he was graduated a bachelor of medicine with honours in 1852; in the same year he became a fellow of the Royal College of Surgeons and house surgeon at University College Hospital. A visit to Edinburgh in the fall of 1853 led to Lister's appointment as assistant to James Syme, the greatest surgical teacher of his day, and in October 1856 he was appointed surgeon to the Edinburgh Royal Infirmary. In April he had married Syme's eldest daughter. Lister, a deeply religious man, joined the Scottish Episcopal Church. The marriage, although childless, was a happy one, his wife entering fully into Lister's professional life.

When three years later the Regius Professorship of Surgery at Glasgow University fell vacant, Lister was elected from seven applicants. In August 1861 he was appointed surgeon to the Glasgow Royal Infirmary, where he was in charge of wards in the new surgical block. The managers hoped that hospital disease (now known as operative sepsis—infection of the blood by disease-producing microorganisms) would be greatly decreased in their new building. The hope proved vain, however. Lister reported that, in his Male Accident Ward, between 45 and 50 percent of his amputation cases died from sepsis between 1861 and 1865.

Work in Antisepsis

In this ward Lister began his experiments with antisepsis. Much of his earlier published work had dealt with the mechanism of coagulation of the blood and role of the blood vessels in the first stages of inflammation. Both researches depended upon the microscope and were directly connected with the healing of wounds. Lister had already tried out methods to encourage clean healing and had formed theories to account for the prevalence of sepsis (a systemic inflammatory condition that occurs as a complication of infection and in severe cases may be associated with acute and life-threatening organ dysfunction). Discarding the popular concept of miasma—direct infection by bad air—he postulated that sepsis might be caused by a pollen-like dust. There is no evidence that he believed this dust to be living matter, but he had come close to the truth. It is therefore all the more surprising that he became acquainted with the work of the bacteriologist Louis Pasteur only in 1865.

Pasteur had arrived at his theory that microorganisms cause fermentation and disease by experiments on fermentation and putrefaction. Lister's education and his familiarity with the microscope, the process of fermentation, and the natural phenomena of inflammation and coagulation of the blood impelled him to accept Pasteur's theory as the full revelation of a half-suspected truth. At the start he believed the germs were carried solely by the air. This incorrect opinion proved useful, for it obliged him to adopt the only feasible method of surgically clean treatment. In his attempt to interpose an antiseptic barrier between the wound and the air, he protected the site of operation from infection by the surgeon's hands and instruments. He found an effective antiseptic in carbolic acid, which had already been used as a means of cleansing foul-smelling sewers and had been empirically advised as a wound dressing in 1863. Lister first successfully used his new method on Aug. 12, 1865; in March 1867 he published a series of cases. The results were dramatic. Between 1865 and 1869, surgical mortality fell from 45 to 15 percent in his Male Accident Ward.

In 1869, Lister succeeded Syme in the chair of Clinical Surgery at Edinburgh. There followed the seven happiest years of his life when, largely as the result of German experiments with antisepsis during the Franco-

German War, his clinics were crowded with visitors and eager students. In 1875 Lister made a triumphal tour of the leading surgical centres in Germany. The next year he visited America but was received with little enthusiasm except in Boston and New York City.

Lister's work had been largely misunderstood in England and the United States. Opposition was directed against his germ theory rather than against his "carbolic treatment." The majority of practicing surgeons were unconvinced; while not antagonistic, they awaited clear proof that antisepsis constituted a major advance. Lister was not a spectacular operative surgeon and refused to publish statistics. Edinburgh, despite the ancient fame of its medical school, was regarded as a provincial centre. Lister understood that he must convince London before the usefulness of his work would be generally accepted.

His chance came in 1877, when he was offered the chair of Clinical Surgery at King's College. On Oct. 26, 1877, Lister, at King's College Hospital, for the first time performed the then-revolutionary operation of wiring a fractured patella, or kneecap. It entailed the deliberate conversion of a simple fracture, carrying no risk to life, into a compound fracture, which often resulted in generalized infection and death. Lister's proposal was widely publicized and aroused much opposition. Thus, the entire success of his operation, which was carried out under antiseptic conditions, forced surgical opinion throughout the world to accept that his method had added greatly to the safety of operative surgery.

More fortunate than many pioneers, Lister saw the almost universal acceptance of his principle during his working life. He retired from surgical practice in 1893, after the death of his wife in the previous year. Many honours came to him. Created a baronet in 1883, he was made

Baron Lister of Lyme Regis in 1897 and appointed one of the 12 original members of the Order of Merit in 1902. He was a gentle, shy, unassuming man, firm in his purpose because he humbly believed himself to be directed by God. He was uninterested in social success or financial reward. In person he was handsome, with a fine athletic figure, fresh complexion, hazel eyes, and silver hair. For some years before his death he was almost completely blind and deaf. Lister wrote no books but contributed many papers to professional journals. These are contained in *The Collected Papers of Joseph, Baron Lister,* 2 vol. (1909).

EMELINE HORTON CLEVELAND
(born Sept. 22, 1829, Ashford, Conn., U.S.–died Dec. 8, 1878, Philadelphia, Pa.)

Emeline Horton Cleveland (née Emeline Horton) was an American physician and college professor. She was widely respected among her male colleagues and served as a strong force for professional opportunity and education for women in medicine.

Horton grew up in Madison County, N.Y. She worked as a teacher until she could afford to enroll at Oberlin (Ohio) College, from which she graduated in 1853. She then entered the Female (later Woman's) Medical College of Pennsylvania in Philadelphia and took her M.D. degree in 1855. While working toward her medical degree she married the Reverend Giles B. Cleveland. Her husband's ill health ended their plan to undertake missionary work, and, after a year of private practice, Cleveland became a demonstrator of anatomy at the Female Medical College. She soon was named professor of anatomy and histology. In 1860–61, with the support of Ann Preston, a doctor at the college, Cleveland took advanced training in obstetrics at the school of the Maternité hospital in Paris. Upon her return to Philadelphia, she became chief resident at the rechartered Woman's Medical College, a post she held until 1868. From 1862 she also taught obstetrics and diseases of women and children and carried on an extensive private practice.

Cleveland's professional reputation was unsurpassed among women physicians. On several occasions she was consulted by male colleagues, and she eventually was admitted to membership in several all-male local medical societies. Her work at the college, where she had early established training courses for nurses and for nurse's aides (the latter a pioneering venture), was capped by her tenure as dean, succeeding Preston, in 1872–74. In 1875, in what was apparently the earliest recorded instance of major surgery performed by a woman, she performed the first of several ovariotomies. In 1878 she was appointed gynecologist to the department for the insane at Pennsylvania Hospital, but she died late that year.

REBECCA LEE CRUMPLER
(born Feb. 8, 1831, Del., U.S.–died March 9, 1895, Fairview, Mass.)

Recognized as the first African American woman to become a physician in the United States, Rebecca Lee Crumpler also holds the distinction of being one of the first African Americans to write a medical book. She published *A Book on Medical Discourses* in 1883.

Born Rebecca Davis, she was primarily raised in Pennsylvania by her aunt. The aunt frequently cared for her sick neighbours, which may have served as an early career influence for Crumpler. By 1852 Crumpler had moved to Charlestown, Mass., where she worked as a nurse for eight years. Her compassion and dedication gained her notice from the doctors she served under, and with their recommendations she was admitted to the New England Female Medical College in Boston, Mass., in 1860. When she graduated four years later, Crumpler was not only the first African American woman in the United States to earn a medical degree but also the only African American woman to graduate from the college (it subsequently merged with Boston University in 1873).

Crumpler started her practice as a general practitioner in Boston. When the Civil War ended in 1865, she moved her practice to Richmond, Va., recognizing the urgent need of medical care among the thousands of newly freed black slaves in the South. While in Richmond, Crumpler worked with numerous black community and missionary groups, as well as with the Freedmen's Bureau. After a number of years, she returned to Boston, establishing a practice and focusing her medical work on the illnesses affecting poor women and children. Her two-volume work, *A Book of Medical Discourses* (1883), was specifically aimed at women and children.

MARY JANE SAFFORD

(born Dec. 31, 1834, Hyde Park, Vt., U.S.–died Dec. 8, 1891, Tarpon Springs, Fla.)

Mary Jane Safford was an American physician whose extensive nursing experience during the Civil War determined her on a medical career. Safford grew up from the age of three in Crete, Ill. During the 1850s she taught school while living with an older brother successively in Joliet, Shawneetown, and Cairo, Ill.

At the outbreak of the Civil War in the spring of 1861, Cairo became a town of some strategic importance because of its situation at the confluence of the Ohio and Mississippi rivers. The town was quickly occupied by volunteer troops from Chicago, and almost as quickly a variety of epidemic diseases broke out in the hastily constructed camps behind the levee. Safford began visiting the camps to tend the sick and to distribute food she had prepared. She gradually won the respect of officers and surgeons who had initially opposed her, and she was soon permitted to draw upon supplies collected and forwarded by the U.S. Sanitary Commission. By summer she was working closely with "Mother" Mary Ann Bickerdyke, who gave her some training in nursing. In November 1861 Safford nursed the wounded on the battlefield at Belmont, Mo. In February 1862 she and Bickerdyke helped transport wounded from Fort Donelson to Cairo, and in April of that year, following the Battle of Shiloh (Pittsburg Landing) in southwestern Tennessee, she worked aboard the hospital ship *Hazel Dell*. By that time her almost ceaseless labours had left her utterly exhausted, and she saw no more service during the war.

After an extended convalescent tour of Europe, Safford returned to the United States determined to become a physician. She graduated from the New York Medical College for Women in 1869 and then pursued advanced training in Europe for three years. At the University of Breslau, Germany (now Wroclaw, Poland), she became the first woman to perform an ovariotomy. In 1872 she opened a private practice in Chicago. The next year, after her marriage to a Bostonian, she moved her practice to that city and became professor of women's diseases at the Boston University School of Medicine and a staff physician at the Massachusetts Homeopathic Hospital. She retired from medical practice in 1886.

MARY PUTNAM JACOBI
(born Aug. 31, 1842, London, England–died June 10, 1906, New York, N.Y., U.S.)

Mary Putnam Jacobi (née Mary Corinna Putnam) was an American physician, writer, and suffragist who is considered to have been the foremost woman doctor of her era.

Mary Putnam was the daughter of George Palmer Putnam, founder of the publishing firm of G.P. Putnam's Sons, and was an elder sister of Herbert Putnam, later librarian of Congress. The family returned from England in 1848, and Mary grew up in Staten Island, Yonkers, and Morrisania, New York. Her scientific bent determined her on a medical career, but in 1860, before she was 18, she had a story published in the *Atlantic Monthly*. She graduated from the New York College of Pharmacy in 1863 and from the Female (later Woman's) Medical College of Pennsylvania in 1864.

After working for a few months at the New England Hospital for Women and Children in Boston, Putnam decided in 1866 to seek further training in Paris. There she attended clinics, lectures, and a class at the École Pratique until she decided to seek admission to the École de Médecine. Her persistence finally secured a directive from the minister of education forcing the faculty to admit her in 1868. Her course was a distinguished one, and she graduated in 1871 with a prizewinning thesis. During her stay in Paris she contributed letters, articles, and stories to the *Medical Record*, *Putnam's Magazine*, the *New York Evening Post*, and *Scribner's Monthly*.

In the fall of 1871 Putnam returned to New York City, opened a practice, and began teaching at Dr. Elizabeth Blackwell's Woman's Medical College of the New York

Infirmary for Women and Children. The quality of her own education had highlighted for her the meagreness of that available to most women aiming for a medical career, and in 1872 she organized the Association for the Advancement of the Medical Education of Women (later the Women's Medical Association of New York City) to begin redressing that shortcoming; she was president of the association from 1874 to 1903. In 1873 she married Dr. Abraham Jacobi, a German-born physician who established the first clinic for diseases of children in the United States (1860) and is generally considered the founder of pediatrics in America. In the same year, Mary Jacobi began a children's dispensary service at Mount Sinai Hospital. From 1882 to 1885 she lectured on diseases of children at the New York Post-Graduate Medical School. She opened a small children's ward at the New York Infirmary in 1886. She resigned her professorship at the Woman's Medical College in 1889 but continued to be a force for improved education for women. From 1893 she was visiting physician at St. Mark's Hospital. In addition to clinical work and teaching, she found time for writing as well.

Jacobi's bibliography runs to more than a hundred titles, mainly in pathology, neurology, pediatrics, and medical education, and one of her essays won the 1876 Boylston Prize from Harvard. Her books include *The Value of Life* (1879), *Essays on Hysteria, Brain-Tumor, and Some Other Cases of Nervous Disease* (1888), *Physiological Notes on Primary Education and the Study of Language* (1889), and *"Common Sense" Applied to Woman Suffrage* (1894). While she did little original research, her contribution to the status of women within the medical profession was incalculable. She also took an interest in social causes. She helped found the Working Women's Society (from 1890 the New York Consumers' League) and the League for Political Education.

ROBERT KOCH

(born Dec. 11, 1843, Clausthal, Hannover [now Clausthal-Zellerfeld, Germany]–died May 27, 1910, Baden-Baden, Germany)

Robert Koch (in full Robert Heinrich Hermann Koch) was a German physician and one of the founders of bacteriology. He discovered the anthrax disease cycle (1876) and the bacteria responsible for tuberculosis (1882) and cholera (1883). For his discoveries in regard to tuberculosis, he received the Nobel Prize for Physiology or Medicine in 1905.

Early Training

Koch attended the University of Göttingen, where he studied medicine, graduating in 1866. He then became a physician in various provincial towns. After serving briefly as a field surgeon during the Franco-Prussian War of 1870–71, he became district surgeon in Wollstein, where he built a small laboratory. Equipped with a microscope, a microtome (an instrument for cutting thin slices of tissue), and a homemade incubator, he began his study of algae, switching later to pathogenic (disease-causing) organisms.

Anthrax Research

One of Koch's teachers at Göttingen had been the anatomist and histologist Friedrich Gustav Jacob Henle, who in 1840 had published the theory that infectious diseases are caused by living microscopic organisms. In 1850 the French parasitologist Casimir Joseph Davaine was among the first to observe organisms in the blood of diseased animals. In 1863 he reported the transmission of anthrax—an acute, infectious, febrile disease of animals and humans—by the inoculation of healthy sheep with the blood of animals dying of the disease and the finding of microscopic rod-shaped bodies in the blood of both groups of sheep. Inspired by the work of the French microbiologist Louis Pasteur, Davaine showed that it was highly probable that, because the sheep did not become diseased in the absence of these rodlike bodies, anthrax was due to the presence of such organisms in the blood. The natural history of the disease was, nevertheless, far from complete.

It was at that point that Koch began. He cultivated the anthrax organisms in suitable media on microscope slides, demonstrated their growth into long filaments, and discovered the formation within them of oval, translucent bodies—dormant spores. Koch found that the dried spores could remain viable for years, even under exposed conditions. The finding explained the recurrence of the disease in pastures long unused for grazing, for the dormant spores could, under the right conditions, develop into the rod-shaped bacteria (bacilli) that cause anthrax. The anthrax life cycle, which Koch had discovered, was announced and illustrated at Breslau in 1876, on the invitation of Ferdinand Cohn, an eminent botanist. Julius Cohnheim, a famous pathologist, was deeply impressed by Koch's presentation. "It leaves nothing more to be proved," he said. "I regard it as the greatest discovery ever made with bacteria and I believe that this is not the last time that this young Robert Koch will surprise and shame us by the brilliance of his investigations."

Cohn, whose discovery of spores had been published in 1875, was also very much impressed and generously helped to prepare the engraving for Koch's epochal paper, which he also published. One of Cohn's pupils, Joseph Schroeter, found that chromogenic (colour-forming) bacteria would grow on such solid substrates as potato, coagulated egg white, meat, and bread and that those colonies were capable of forming new colonies of the same colour, consisting of organisms of the same type. That was the starting point of Koch's pure-culture techniques, which he worked out a few years later. That a disease organism might be cultured outside the body was a concept introduced by Louis Pasteur, but the pure-culture techniques for doing so were perfected by Koch, whose precise and ingenious experiments demonstrated the complete life cycle of an important organism. The anthrax work afforded for the first time convincing proof of the definite causal relation of a particular microorganism to a particular disease.

Contributions to General Bacteriology and Pathology

In 1877 Koch published an important paper on the investigation, preservation, and photographing of bacteria. His work was illustrated by superb photomicrographs. In his paper he described his method of preparing thin layers of bacteria on glass slides and fixing them by gentle heat. Koch also invented the apparatus and the procedure for the very useful hanging-drop technique, whereby microorganisms could be cultured in a drop of nutrient solution on the underside of a glass slide.

In 1878 Koch summarized his experiments on the etiology of wound infection. By inoculating animals with material from various sources, he produced six types of infection, each caused by a specific microorganism. He then transferred these infections by inoculation through several kinds of animals, reproducing the original six types. In that study, he observed differences in pathogenicity for different species of hosts and demonstrated that the animal body is an excellent apparatus for the cultivation of bacteria.

Koch, now recognized as a scientific investigator of the first rank, obtained a position in Berlin in the Imperial Health Office, where he set up a laboratory in bacteriology. With his collaborators, he devised new research methods to isolate pathogenic bacteria. Koch determined guidelines to prove that a disease is caused by a specific organism. These four basic criteria, called Koch's postulates, are:

- A specific microorganism is always associated with a given disease.
- The microorganism can be isolated from the diseased animal and grown in pure culture in the laboratory.
- The cultured microbe will cause disease when transferred to a healthy animal.
- The same type of microorganism can be isolated from the newly infected animal.

Studies of Tuberculosis and Cholera

Koch concentrated his efforts on the study of tuberculosis, with the aim of isolating its cause. Although it was suspected that tuberculosis was caused by an infectious agent, the organism had not yet been isolated and identified. By modifying the method of staining, Koch discovered the tubercle bacillus and established its presence in the tissues of animals and humans suffering from the disease. A fresh difficulty arose when for some time it proved impossible to grow the organism in pure culture. But eventually Koch succeeded in isolating the organism in a succession of media and induced tuberculosis in animals by inoculating them with it. Its etiologic role was thereby established. On March 24, 1882, Koch announced before the Physiological Society of Berlin that he had isolated and grown the tubercle bacillus, which he believed to be the cause of all forms of tuberculosis.

Meanwhile, Koch's work was interrupted by an outbreak of cholera in Egypt and the danger of its transmission to Europe. As a member of a German government commission, Koch went to Egypt to investigate the disease. Although he soon had reason to suspect a particular comma-shaped bacterium (vibrio) as the cause of cholera, the epidemic ended before he was able to confirm his hypothesis. Nevertheless, he raised awareness of amebic dysentery and differentiated two varieties of Egyptian conjunctivitis.

Proceeding to India, where cholera is endemic, he completed his task, identifying both the organism responsible for the disease and its transmission via drinking water, food, and clothing. By employing a technique he invented of inoculating sterilized gelatin-coated glass plates with fecal material from patients, he was able to grow and describe the bacterium. He was then able to show that its presence in a person's intestine led to the development of cholera in that person.

Koch's findings, however, were not original. Rather, they were rediscoveries of work that had been previously done by others. The Italian microbiologist Filippo Pacini had already seen the bacterium and named it "cholerigenic vibrios" in 1854 (a fact of which Koch is assumed not to have been aware). The principal mode of cholera transmission, contaminated water, had also been described previously—by the British anesthesiologist John Snow in 1849. Snow's work, however, was not totally accepted at the time, since other theories of disease causation were prevalent, most notably that of "miasmatism," which claimed that cholera was contracted by breathing air contaminated by disease-containing "clouds."

Resuming his studies of tuberculosis, Koch investigated the effect an injection of dead bacilli had on a person who subsequently received a dose of living bacteria and concluded that he may have discovered a cure for the disease. In his studies he used as the active agent a sterile liquid produced from cultures of the bacillus. However, the liquid, which he named tuberculin (1890), proved disappointing, and sometimes dangerous, as a curative agent. Consequently, its importance as a means of detecting a present or past tubercular state was not immediately recognized. Additional work on tuberculosis came later, but, after the seeming debacle of tuberculin, Koch was also occupied with a great variety of investigations into diseases of humans and animals—studies of leprosy, bubonic plague, livestock diseases, and malaria.

In 1901 Koch reported work done on the pathogenicity of the human tubercle bacillus in domestic animals. He believed that infection of human beings by bovine tuberculosis is so rare that it is not necessary to take any measures against it. That conclusion was rejected by commissions of inquiry in Europe and America but extensive and important work was stimulated by Koch. As a result, successful measures of prophylaxis were devised.

Historical Assessment

Not an eloquent speaker, Koch was nevertheless by example, demonstration, and precept one of the most effective of teachers, and his numerous pupils—from the entire Western world and Asia—were the creators of the new era of bacteriology. His work on trypanosomes was of direct use to the eminent German bacteriologist Paul Ehrlich; that is only one example of Koch's instigation of epochal work both within and beyond his own immediate sphere.

His discoveries and his technical innovations were matched by his fundamental concepts of the etiology of disease. Long before his death, his place in the history of science was universally recognized.

WILHELM CONRAD RÖNTGEN
(born March 27, 1845, Lennep, Prussia [now Remscheid, Germany]– died Feb. 10, 1923, Munich, Germany)

Wilhelm Röntgen (also spelled Roentgen) was a physicist who received the first Nobel Prize for Physics, in 1901, for his discovery of X-rays, which heralded the age of modern physics and revolutionized diagnostic medicine.

Röntgen studied at the Polytechnic in Zürich and then was professor of physics at the universities of Strasbourg (1876–79), Giessen (1879–88), Würzburg (1888–1900), and Munich (1900–20). His research also included work on elasticity, capillary action of fluids, specific heats of gases, conduction of heat in crystals, absorption of heat by gases, and piezoelectricity.

In 1895, while experimenting with electric current flow in a partially evacuated glass tube (cathode-ray tube), Röntgen observed that a nearby piece of barium platinocyanide gave off light when the tube was in operation. He theorized that when the cathode rays (electrons) struck the glass wall of the tube, some unknown radiation was formed that traveled across the room, struck the chemical, and caused the fluorescence. Further investigation revealed that paper, wood, and aluminum, among other materials, are transparent to this new form of radiation. He found that it affected photographic plates, and, since it did not noticeably exhibit any properties of light, such as reflection or refraction, he mistakenly thought the rays were unrelated to light. In view of its uncertain nature, he called the phenomenon X-radiation, though it also became known as Röntgen radiation. He took the first X-ray photographs, of the interiors of metal objects and of the bones in his wife's hand.

Within months of the discovery there was an extensive literature on the subject: Robert Jones, a British surgeon, had localized a bullet in a boy's wrist before operating; stones in the urinary bladder and gallbladder had been demonstrated; and fractures had been displayed.

ALPHONSE LAVERAN
(born June 18, 1845, Paris, France–died May 18, 1922, Paris)

Alphonse Laveran (in full Charles-Louis-Alphonse Laveran) was a French physician, pathologist, and parasitologist who discovered the parasite that causes human malaria. For this and later work on protozoal diseases he received the Nobel Prize for Physiology or Medicine in 1907.

Educated at the Strasbourg faculty of medicine, he served as an army surgeon in the Franco-German War (1870–71) and practiced and taught military medicine until 1897, when he joined the Pasteur Institute, Paris. While serving as a military surgeon in Algeria in 1880, Laveran discovered the cause of malaria in the course of the autopsies he conducted on malaria victims. He found the causative organism to be a protozoan which he named *Oscillaria malariae,* though it was later renamed *Plasmodium.*

Malarial fevers were associated with swamps and marshes as early as classical Greece, but the role of mosquitoes in transmitting the infection was completely unknown. Many of the early Greeks thought the disease was contracted by drinking swamp water; later, because the Romans attributed it to breathing "miasmas," or vapours, arising from bodies of stagnant water, the disease came to be called *mal aria*, or "bad air." Since early Greek times, attempts were made to control malaria by draining swamps and stagnant marshes, but a specific treatment for the disease did not become available in Europe until the 1630s, when bark of the cinchona tree was introduced into Spain from Peru. The skillful use of "Peruvian bark" by the great English physician Thomas Sydenham helped to separate malaria from other fevers and served as one of the first practices of specific drug therapy. The lifesaving drug became much more widely available by the mid-19th century, after the active ingredient of cinchona, quinine, was successfully isolated and the Dutch began to cultivate the cinchona tree in plantations on the island of Java.

Following the introduction of cinchona bark, no comparably significant advance in the understanding of malaria or its control came until after the 1870s, when pioneering studies by Louis Pasteur in France and Robert Koch in Germany laid the foundations of modern microbiology. Laveran, showed that the elements seen in red blood cells of certain patients were parasites responsible for their hosts' malaria.

Laveran was a powerful influence in developing research in tropical medicine, carrying on fruitful work in trypanosomiasis, leishmaniasis, and other protozoal diseases, as well as his epochal work in malaria. He established the Laboratory of Tropical Diseases at the Pasteur Institute (1907) and founded the Société de Pathologie Exotique (1908).

Laveran's extensive writings include *Trypanosomes et trypanosomiasis* (with Félix Mesnil; 1904); *Traité des fièvres palustres avec la description des microbes du paludisme* (1884); and *Traité des maladies et épidémies des armées* (1875).

WILLIAM OSLER

(born July 12, 1849, Bond Head, Canada West [now Ontario], Canada–died Dec. 29, 1919, Oxford, England)

William Osler was a Canadian physician and professor of medicine who practiced and taught in Canada, the United States, and Great Britain and whose book *The Principles and Practice of Medicine* (1892) was a leading textbook. Osler played a key role in transforming the organization and curriculum of medical education, emphasizing the importance of clinical experience. He was created a baronet in 1911.

William Osler was the youngest of the nine children of the Reverend Featherstone Osler, who had gone to Canada as an Anglican missionary, and his wife, Ellen. William, like his father, was intended for the church. But while at school he became fascinated by natural history. He began to study at Trinity College, Toronto, but decided that the church was not for him and entered the Toronto Medical School in 1868. He subsequently transferred to McGill University in Montreal, Que., where he took his medical degree in 1872. During the following two years he visited medical centres in Europe, spending the longest period at University College, London, in the physiology laboratory of John Burdon-Sanderson, who was making experimental physiology preeminent in medical education.

In 1873 Osler demonstrated that hitherto unidentified bodies in the blood were in fact the third kind of blood corpuscles, which were later named the blood platelets. These corpuscles had been observed before, but no one before Osler had studied them so thoroughly. Thus began what he called his periods of "brain dusting"—travel and studies that made him almost as much a part of Europe as of America.

Osler returned to Canada and began general practice in Dundas but was soon appointed lecturer in the institutes of medicine at McGill University. He became professor there in 1875. A year later he became pathologist to the Montreal General Hospital and in 1878 physician to that hospital. At McGill he taught physiology, pathology, and medicine. His research was conducted largely in the postmortem room. In 1884 he was invited to occupy the chair of clinical medicine at the University of Pennsylvania in Philadelphia. He decided to do so on the toss of a coin. While in Philadelphia he became a founding member of the Association of American Physicians.

In 1888 Osler became the first professor of medicine in the new Johns Hopkins University Medical School in Baltimore. There he joined William H. Welch, chief of pathology, Howard A. Kelly, chief of gynecology and obstetrics, and William S. Halsted, chief of surgery. Together, the four transformed the organization and curriculum of clinical teaching and made Johns Hopkins the most famous medical school in the world. Students studied their patients in the wards and presented the results to the "Chief." They were also encouraged to take their problems to the laboratory. Finally, the experts pooled their knowledge for the benefit of the patient and the student in public teaching sessions. Thus was born the pattern of clinical teaching that spread throughout the United States. Osler was not only professor of medicine but physician in chief to the hospital, an office first devised by the president of the university on the basis of his experience of running a large department store and later to spread to most of the medical centres of the United States. For the first four years there were no students at Johns Hopkins, and Osler used the time to write *The Principles and Practice of Medicine,* first published in 1892. In the same year, he married Grace Gross, widow of a surgical colleague at Philadelphia and great-granddaughter of Paul Revere.

Osler's textbook was lucid, comprehensive, interesting, and scholarly. It quickly became the most popular medical textbook of its day and has continued to be published since under a succession of editors, though never regaining the quality with which Osler endowed it. The textbook had an unexpected sequel. In 1897 it was read by F.T. Gates, who had been engaged by John D. Rockefeller to advise him in his philanthropic endeavours. As a result of his reading, Gates inspired Rockefeller to direct his foundation toward medical research and to establish the Rockefeller Institute of Medical Research in New York.

In 1904, while visiting in England, Osler was invited to succeed Sir John Burdon-Sanderson in the Regius chair of medicine at the University of Oxford. Osler's practice and teaching had for many years imposed enormous demands on his time and energy. His forceful wife telegraphed him from America: "Do not procrastinate. Accept at once." Osler did. The Regius chair at Oxford is a crown appointment for which only citizens of the crown are eligible, but Osler had kept his Canadian nationality. He took up his chair in the autumn of 1905. In Oxford he taught only once a week, did a small amount of practice, and spent most of his time on his books. His library became one of the best of its kind, and after his death it passed intact to McGill, where it is specially housed. His scholarship was recognized by his election as president of the Classical Association. He was also active in medical affairs and inspired the formation of the Association of Physicians of Great Britain and Ireland and the establishment of the *Quarterly Journal of Medicine*. He was elected a fellow of the Royal College of Physicians of London in 1884 and a fellow of the Royal Society of London in 1898. He and his wife were immensely hospitable, especially to visiting Americans, among whom their house was known as the "Open Arms."

Osler gave many lectures on medicine, some of which were collected and published. *Aequanimitas,* which he regarded as the most desirable quality for doctors, was the title of the most famous of these. Osler had a puckish wit and wrote some admirable medical nonsense under the pseudonym of Egerton Yorrick Davis, whom he presented as a retired surgeon captain of the U.S. Army.

In medical terminology, Osler is immortalized in Osler's nodes (red, tender swellings of the hand characteristic of certain cardiac infections), a blood disorder known as Osler-Vaquez disease, and Osler-Rendu-Weber disease (a hereditary disorder marked by recurring nose bleeds with vascular involvement of the skin and mucous membranes).

The Oslers had one son, Revere, named after his great-great-grandfather, Paul Revere. His death in action during World War I took the spirit out of his father, who died of pneumonia in 1919.

WALTER REED

(born Sept.13, 1851, Belroi, Va., U.S.–died Nov. 22, 1902, Washington, D.C.)

Walter Reed was a U.S. Army pathologist and bacteriologist who led the experiments that proved that yellow fever is transmitted by the bite of a mosquito. The Walter Reed Hospital, Washington, D.C., was named in his honour.

Reed was the youngest of five children of Lemuel Sutton Reed, a Methodist minister, and his first wife, Pharaba White. In 1866 the family moved to Charlottesville, where Walter intended to study classics at the University of Virginia. After a period at the university he transferred to the medical faculty, completed his

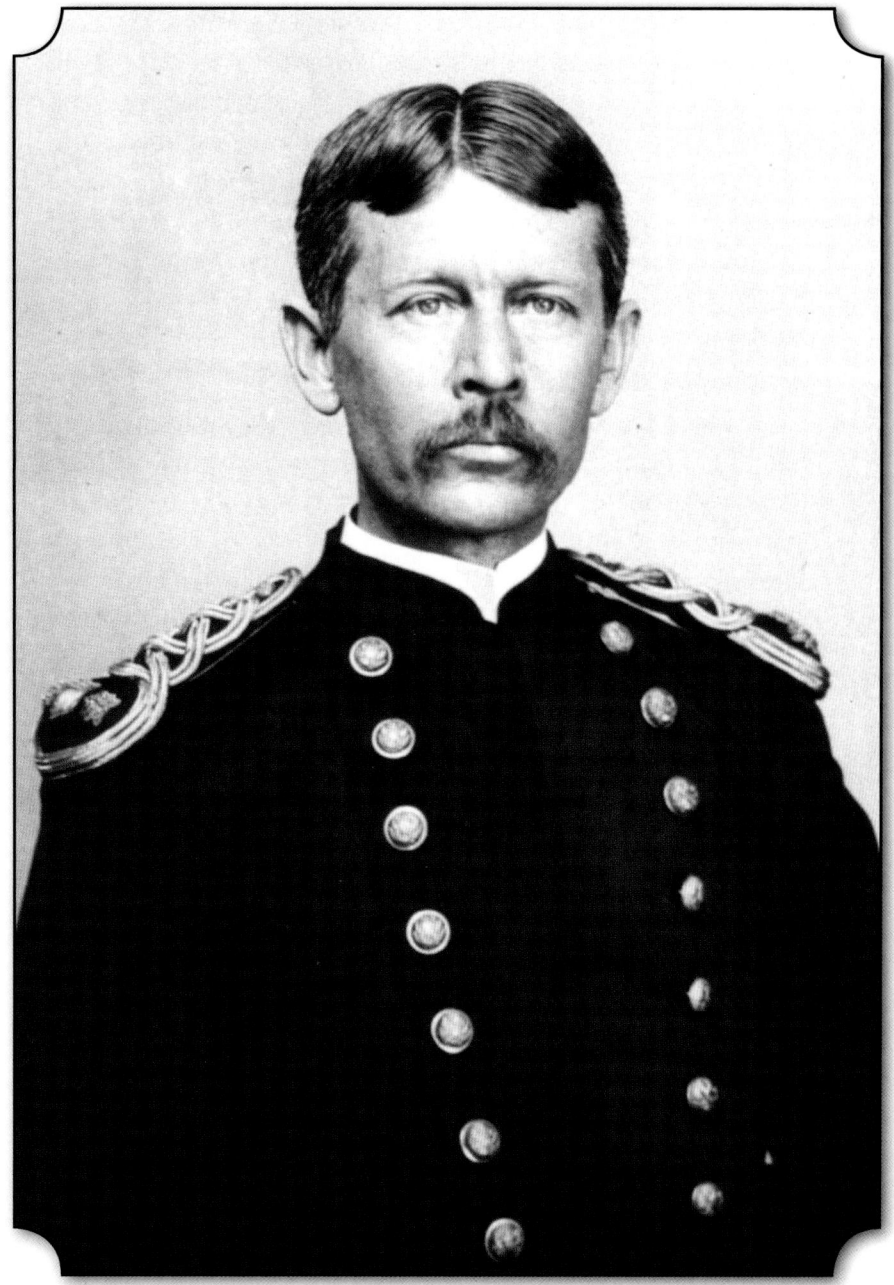

American physician Walter Reed proved that yellow fever, like malaria, was also transmitted by mosquitoes.

medical course in nine months, and in the summer of 1869, at the age of 17, was graduated as a doctor of medicine. To obtain further clinical experience, he matriculated as a medical student at Bellevue Medical College, New York, and a year later took a second medical degree there. He held several hospital posts as an intern and was a district physician in New York. He decided against general practice, however, and for security chose a military career. In February 1875 he passed the examination for the Army Medical Corps and was commissioned a first lieutenant.

After marrying Emilie Lawrence in April 1876, Reed was transferred to Fort Lowell in Arizona, where his wife soon joined him. During the next 18 years—changing stations almost every year—Reed was on garrison duty, often at frontier stations. His letters provide vivid pictures of the rigours of frontier life. In 1889 he was appointed attending surgeon and examiner of recruits at Baltimore. He had permission to work at the Johns Hopkins Hospital, where he took courses in pathology and bacteriology. In 1893 Reed was assigned to the posts of curator of the Army Medical Museum in Washington and of professor of bacteriology and clinical microscopy at the newly established Army Medical School. During the Spanish-American War of 1898 he was appointed chairman of a committee to investigate the spread of typhoid fever in military camps. Its report, not published until 1904, revealed new facts regarding this disease. On the completion of the committee's work in 1899, he returned to his duties in Washington. Almost immediately he became involved in the problem of yellow fever. The result was a brilliant investigation in epidemiology.

During most of the 19th century it had been widely held that yellow fever was spread by fomites—i.e., articles such as bedding and clothing that had been used by a yellow-fever patient. As late as 1898 a U.S. official report ascribed the spread to this cause. Meanwhile, other methods of transmission had been suggested. In 1881 the Cuban physician and epidemiologist Carlos Juan Finlay began to formulate a theory of insect transmission. In succeeding years he maintained and developed the theory but did not succeed in proving it. In 1896 an Italian bacteriologist, Giuseppe Sanarelli, claimed that he had isolated from yellow-fever patients an organism he called *Bacillus icteroides*. The U.S. Army now appointed Reed and army physician James Carroll to investigate Sanarelli's bacillus. It also sent Aristides Agramonte, an assistant surgeon in the U.S. Army, to investigate the yellow-fever cases in Cuba. Agramonte isolated Sanarelli's bacillus not only from one-third of the yellow-fever patients but also from persons suffering from other diseases. Reed and Carroll published their first report in April 1899 and in February 1900 submitted a complete report for publication. It showed that Sanarelli's bacillus belonged to the group of the hog-cholera bacillus and was in yellow fever a secondary invader.

Before this report had actually been published, an outbreak of yellow fever occurred in the U.S. garrison at Havana, and a commission was appointed to investigate it. The members of the commission were Reed, who was to act as chairman, Carroll, Agramonte, and a bacteriologist, Jesse W. Lazear. In the summer of 1900, when the commission investigated an outbreak of what had been diagnosed as malaria in barracks 200 miles (300 kilometres) from Havana, Reed found that the disease was actually yellow fever. Of the nine prisoners in the prison cell of the post, one contracted yellow fever and died, but none of the other eight was affected.

Reed and his colleagues thought it possible that this patient, and only he, might have been bitten by some insect. Reed therefore decided that the main work of the commission would be to prove or disprove the agency of an insect intermediate host.

On Aug. 27, 1900, an infected mosquito was allowed to feed on Carroll, and he developed a severe attack of yellow fever. Shortly afterward Lazear was bitten, developed yellow fever, and died. In November 1900 a small hutted camp was established, and controlled experiments were performed on volunteers. Reed proved that an attack of yellow fever was caused by the bite of an infected mosquito, *Stegomyia fasciata* (later renamed *Aedes aegypti*), and that the same result could be obtained by injecting into a volunteer blood drawn from a patient suffering from yellow fever. Reed found no evidence that yellow fever could be conveyed by fomites, and he showed that a house became infected only by the presence of infected mosquitoes. In February 1901 official action in Cuba was begun by U.S. military engineers under Major W.C. Gorgas on the basis of Reed's findings, and within 90 days Havana was freed from yellow fever.

On his return to Washington in February 1901, Reed continued his teaching duties. He died following an operation for appendicitis the next year.

SANTIAGO RAMÓN Y CAJAL

(born May 1, 1852, Petilla de Aragón, Spain–died Oct. 17, 1934, Madrid)

Santiago Ramón y Cajal was a Spanish histologist who (with Camillo Golgi) received the 1906 Nobel Prize for Physiology or Medicine for establishing the neuron, or nerve cell, as the basic unit of nervous structure. This finding was instrumental in the recognition of the neuron's fundamental role in nervous function and in gaining a modern understanding of the nerve impulse.

Ramón y Cajal obtained a medical degree at the University of Zaragoza in 1873 and became an assistant in the medical faculty there two years later. He served as professor of descriptive anatomy at the University of Valencia (1884–87) and professor of histology and pathological anatomy at the universities of Barcelona (1887–92) and Madrid (1892–1922). He improved Golgi's silver nitrate stain (1903) and developed a gold stain (1913) for the general study of the fine structure of nervous tissue in the brain, sensory centres, and the spinal cords of embryos and young animals. These nerve-specific stains enabled Ramón y Cajal to differentiate neurons from other cells and to trace the structure and connections of nerve cells in gray matter and the spinal cord. The stains have also been of great value in the diagnosis of brain tumours.

In 1920 King Alfonso XIII of Spain commissioned the construction of the Cajal Institute in Madrid, where Ramón y Cajal worked until his death. Among his many books concerning nervous structure is *Estudios sobre la degeneración y regeneración del sistema nervioso,* 2 vol. (1913–14; *The Degeneration and Regeneration of the Nervous System*).

KITASATO SHIBASABURO

(born Jan. 29, 1853, Kitanosato, Higo province [now Kumamoto prefecture], Japan–died June 13, 1931, Tokyo)

Kitasato Shibasaburo (also spelled Kitazato Shibasaburo) was a Japanese physician and bacteriologist who helped discover a method to prevent tetanus and diphtheria and, in the same year as Alexandre Yersin, discovered the infectious agent responsible for the bubonic plague.

Kitasato began his study of medicine at Igakusho Hospital (now Kumamoto Medical School). When his mentor, Dutch physician C.G. van Mansvelt, left the school, Kitasato entered Tokyo Medical School (now the Faculty of Medicine, University of Tokyo). After graduation (M.D., 1883) he carried out bacteriological research at the Central Sanitary Bureau of the Ministry of Home Affairs.

In 1885 Kitasato moved to Berlin to join the laboratory of German bacteriologist Robert Koch. There, with Emil von Behring, he studied tetanus and diphtheria, two bacterial infections that cause symptoms through the secretion of toxins. In 1889 Kitasato succeeded in obtaining the first pure culture of the tetanus bacteria (bacilli), and the following year he and von Behring demonstrated that immunity to tetanus could be achieved by injecting a susceptible animal with serum containing antitoxin produced in the blood of an animal exposed to the bacterial toxin. They soon successfully applied this approach, called serum therapy, to the treatment of diphtheria.

Returning to Japan in 1892, Kitasato founded and became president of the Institute for Infectious Diseases, a laboratory near Tokyo that was incorporated in 1899 into the Ministry of Home Affairs. The next year he founded Yojoen, a sanatorium for victims of tuberculosis, and concurrently served as president of both organizations.

Kitasato was sent to Hong Kong in 1894 to investigate an outbreak of the bubonic plague. Within a month he identified the causative organism of the plague, the bacillus *Pasteurella pestis*, now called *Yersinia pestis*; renamed after French bacteriologist Alexandre Yersin, who independently discovered the plague bacillus during the Hong

Kong epidemic. Both men found bacteria in fluid samples taken from plague victims, then injected them into animals and observed that the animals died quickly of plague.

In 1914 Kitasato resigned the directorship of the imperial institute and founded the Kitasato Institute. He became the first dean of the medical school of Keio University, an institution he helped establish, in 1917 and held this position until 1928. When the Japanese Medical Association was founded in 1923, he became its first president. In 1924 the emperor invested him with the title of baron.

PAUL EHRLICH

(born March 14, 1854, Strehlen, Silesia, Prussia [now Strzelin, Poland]–died Aug. 20, 1915, Bad Homburg vor der Höhe, Germany)

Paul Ehrlich was a German medical scientist known for his pioneering work in hematology, immunology, and chemotherapy and for his discovery of the first effective treatment for syphilis. He received jointly with Élie Metchnikoff the Nobel Prize for Physiology or Medicine in 1908.

Early Life

Ehrlich was born into a Jewish family prominent in business and industry. Although he lacked formal training in experimental chemistry and applied bacteriology, he was introduced by his mother's cousin, the pathologist Carl Weigert, to the technique of staining cells with chemical dyes, a procedure used to view cells under the microscope. As a medical student at several universities, including Breslau, Strasbourg, Freiburg, and Leipzig, Ehrlich continued to experiment with cellular staining. The selective action of these dyes on different types of cells suggested to Ehrlich that chemical reactions were occurring in cells and that these reactions formed the basis of cellular processes. From this idea he reasoned that chemical agents could be used to heal diseased cells or to destroy infectious agents, a theory that revolutionized medical diagnostics and therapeutics.

After receiving his medical degree from the University of Leipzig in 1878, Ehrlich was offered a position as head physician at the prestigious Charité Hospital in Berlin. There he developed a new staining technique to identify the tuberculosis bacillus (a bacterium) that had been discovered by the German bacteriologist Robert Koch. Ehrlich also differentiated the numerous types of blood cells of the body and thereby laid the foundation for the field of hematology.

While developing new methods for the staining of live tissue, Ehrlich discovered the uses of methylene blue in the treatment of nervous disorders. In other diagnostic advances, he traced a specific chemical reaction in the urine of typhoid patients, tested various medications for reducing or removing fever, and made valuable suggestions for the treatment of eye diseases. Of the 37 scientific contributions that he published between 1879 and 1885, Ehrlich considered the last as the most important: *Das Sauerstoff-Bedürfniss des Organismus* (1885; "The Requirement of the Organism for Oxygen"). In it he established that oxygen consumption varies with different types of tissue and that these variations constitute a measure of the intensity of vital cell processes.

In 1883 Ehrlich married Hedwig Pinkus, with whom he had two daughters.

IMMUNITY AND THE SIDE-CHAIN THEORY

A bout with tuberculosis forced Ehrlich to interrupt his work and seek a cure in Egypt. When he returned to Berlin in 1889, the disease had been permanently arrested. After working for some time in a tiny and primitive private laboratory, he transferred to Koch's Institute for Infectious Diseases, where he concentrated on the problem of immunity. Very little was known at the time about the precise manner in which bacteria bring about disease, and even less was known about the body's defenses against infection or how these immune defenses could be enhanced. The hypothesis Ehrlich developed to explain immunological phenomena was the side-chain theory, which described how antibodies—the protective proteins produced by the immune system—are formed and how they react with other substances. Delivered to the Royal Society in 1900, this theory was based on an understanding of the way in which a cell was thought to absorb and assimilate nutrients. Ehrlich postulated that each cell has on its surface a series of side chains, or receptors, that function by attaching to certain food molecules. While each side chain interacts with a specific nutrient—in the same manner as a key fits into a lock—it also can interact with other molecules, such as disease-causing toxins (antigens) produced by an infectious agent. When a toxin binds to a side chain, the interaction is irreversible and blocks subsequent binding and uptake of nutrients. The body then tries to overwhelm the obstruction by producing a great number of replacement side chains—so many that they cannot fit on the surface of the cell and instead are secreted into the circulation. According to Ehrlich's theory, these circulating side chains are the antibodies, which are all gauged to and able to neutralize the disease-causing toxin and then remain in the circulation, thus immunizing the individual against subsequent invasions by the infectious agent.

This much-debated hypothesis, although ultimately proven to be incorrect in many particulars, had a profound influence on Ehrlich's later work and on the work of his successors. Thus Ehrlich was able to show experimentally that rabbits subjected to a slow and measured increase of toxic matter were able to survive 5,000 times the fatal dose. In the end, he established precise quantitative patterns of immunity. These findings assumed great importance in 1890, when he met Emil von Behring, who had succeeded in creating an antitoxin against diphtheria. Behring had tried to prepare a serum that could be used in clinical practice, but it was only by adopting Ehrlich's technique of using the blood of live horses that the preparation of a serum of optimum antitoxic effectiveness became possible. Ehrlich developed a way of measuring the effectiveness of serums that was soon adopted all over the world for the standardization of diphtheria serum. He also demonstrated, in 1892, that antibodies are passed in breast milk from mother to newborn.

On the basis of these achievements, Ehrlich was made director of a government-supported institute near Berlin, which was transferred to Frankfurt am Main in 1899 as the Royal Institute for Experimental Therapy. No restrictions of any kind were placed upon the direction of his research. While this corresponded to Ehrlich's own talents and inclinations, it did not please Behring, who endeavoured to have his colleague specialize in immunology and serum therapy. The strained relationship between the two men was exacerbated by personality differences. Ehrlich, utterly indifferent to monetary rewards, had no ambition to become an industrialist like Behring; he was content to carry out his research.

He had by then recognized the limitations of serum therapy. Many infectious disorders, in particular those caused by protozoa rather than bacteria, failed to respond to serum treatment. The recognition of this fact marks the birth of chemotherapy. Ehrlich started experimenting with the identification and synthesis of substances, not necessarily found in nature, that could kill parasites or inhibit their growth without damaging the organism. He began with

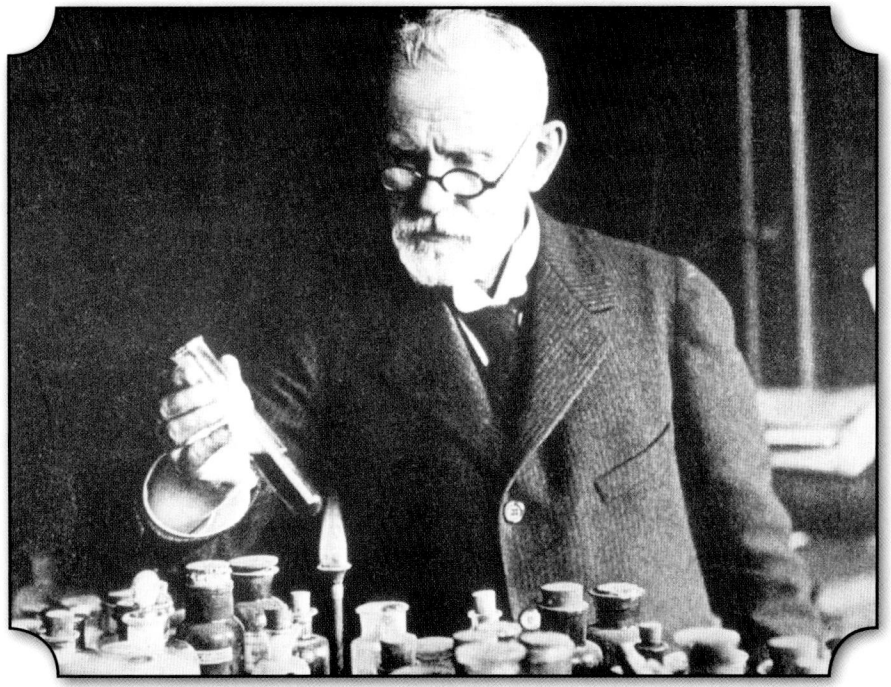

Chemotherapy, as developed by Paul Ehrlich, was originally used against infectious microbes. It is now used to treat many illnesses, including cancer.

trypanosomes, a species of protozoa that he unsuccessfully attempted to control by means of coal tar dyes. There followed compounds of arsenic and benzene; other compounds proved to be too toxic. Instead of declaring himself vanquished by these difficulties, Ehrlich turned his attention to the spirochete *Treponema pallidum*, the causal organism of syphilis.

SYPHILIS STUDIES

Ehrlich had at this time several institutes at his disposal as well as sizable research funds. He also had a staff of highly competent collaborators; in fact, his colleague Hata Sahachiro contributed much to his eventual success in combating syphilis. His preparation 606, later called Salvarsan, was extraordinarily effective and harmless despite its large arsenic content. The first tests, announced in the spring of 1910, proved to be surprisingly successful in the treatment of a whole spectrum of diseases; in the case of yaws, a tropical disease akin to syphilis, a single injection was sufficient. It seemed as if a "magic bullet," to use a favourite expression of Ehrlich's, had been found.

The devastation wrought by syphilis provoked worldwide demand for a new weapon against the disease. Ehrlich, however, would not yet release his discovery for general use, believing as he did that the usual few hundred clinical tests did not suffice in the case of an arsenic preparation, the injection of which required special precautions. In an unheard-of transaction, the manufacturer with whom Ehrlich had collaborated closely, Farbwerke-Hoechst, released a total of 65,000 units gratis to physicians all over the globe. Although harmful side effects remained nominal in number, some envious competitors did not hesitate to attack Ehrlich. The most libelous among them was given a jail sentence.

The greatest distinction bestowed on Ehrlich by the Prussian state was the title "Wirklicher Geheimer Rat," or Privy Councillor, with the predicate of "Exzellenz." Along with numerous other honours, Ehrlich was presented with honorary doctorates by the Universities of Oxford, Chicago, and Athens and an honorary citizenship by Frankfurt am Main, where the institute he founded still bears his name. Having suffered a first stroke in December 1914, Ehrlich succumbed to a second stroke in August of the following year. In its obituary the London *Times* acknowledged Ehrlich's achievement in opening new doors into the unknown, saying, "The whole world is in his debt."

EMIL VON BEHRING
(born March 15, 1854, Hansdorf, West Prussia [now Jankowa Zaganska, Poland]–died March 31, 1917, Marburg, Germany)

Emil von Behring (in full Emil Adolf von Behring) was a German bacteriologist who was one of the founders of immunology. In 1901 he received the first Nobel Prize for Physiology or Medicine for his work on serum therapy, particularly for its use in the treatment of diphtheria.

Behring received his medical degree in 1878 from the Friedrich-Wilhelms-Institut, the Prussian army's medical college, in Berlin. After serving 10 years with the Army Medical Corps, he became an assistant (1889) at the Institute for Hygiene, Berlin, where Robert Koch was director. There, with the Japanese bacteriologist Kitasato Shibasaburo, he showed that it was possible to provide an animal with passive immunity against tetanus by injecting it with the blood serum of another animal infected with the disease. Behring applied this antitoxin (a term he and Kitasato originated) technique to achieve immunity against diphtheria. Administration of diphtheria antitoxin, developed with Paul Ehrlich and first successfully marketed in 1892, became a routine part of the treatment of the disease.

Behring taught at Halle (1894) and in 1895 moved on to become director of the Institute of Hygiene at the Philipps University of Marburg. He became financially involved with the Farbwerke Meister, Lucius und Brüning in Höchst, a dye works that provided laboratories for his research, which included studies of tuberculosis. His writings include *Die praktischen Ziele der Blutserumtherapie* (1892; "The Practical Goals of Blood Serum Therapy").

SIGMUND FREUD

(born May 6, 1856, Freiberg, Moravia, Austrian Empire [now Příbor, Czech Republic]–died Sept. 23, 1939, London, England)

Sigmund Freud, an Austrian neurologist, was the founder of psychoanalysis. Freud may justly be called the most influential intellectual legislator of his age. His creation of psychoanalysis was at once a theory of the human psyche, a therapy for the relief of its ills, and an optic for the interpretation of culture and society. Despite repeated criticisms, attempted refutations, and qualifications of Freud's work, its spell remained powerful well after his death and in fields far removed from psychology as it is narrowly defined. If, as the American sociologist Philip Rieff once contended, "psychological man" replaced such earlier notions as political, religious, or economic man as the 20th century's dominant self-image, it is in no small measure due to the power of Freud's vision and the seeming inexhaustibility of the intellectual legacy he left behind.

EARLY LIFE AND TRAINING

Freud's father, Jakob, was a Jewish wool merchant who had been married once before he wed the boy's mother, Amalie Nathansohn. Hia father, 40 years old at Freud's birth, seems to have been a relatively remote and authoritarian figure, while his mother appears to have been more nurturant and emotionally available. Although Freud had two older half-brothers, his strongest if also most ambivalent attachment seems to have been to a nephew, John, one

Sigmund Freud

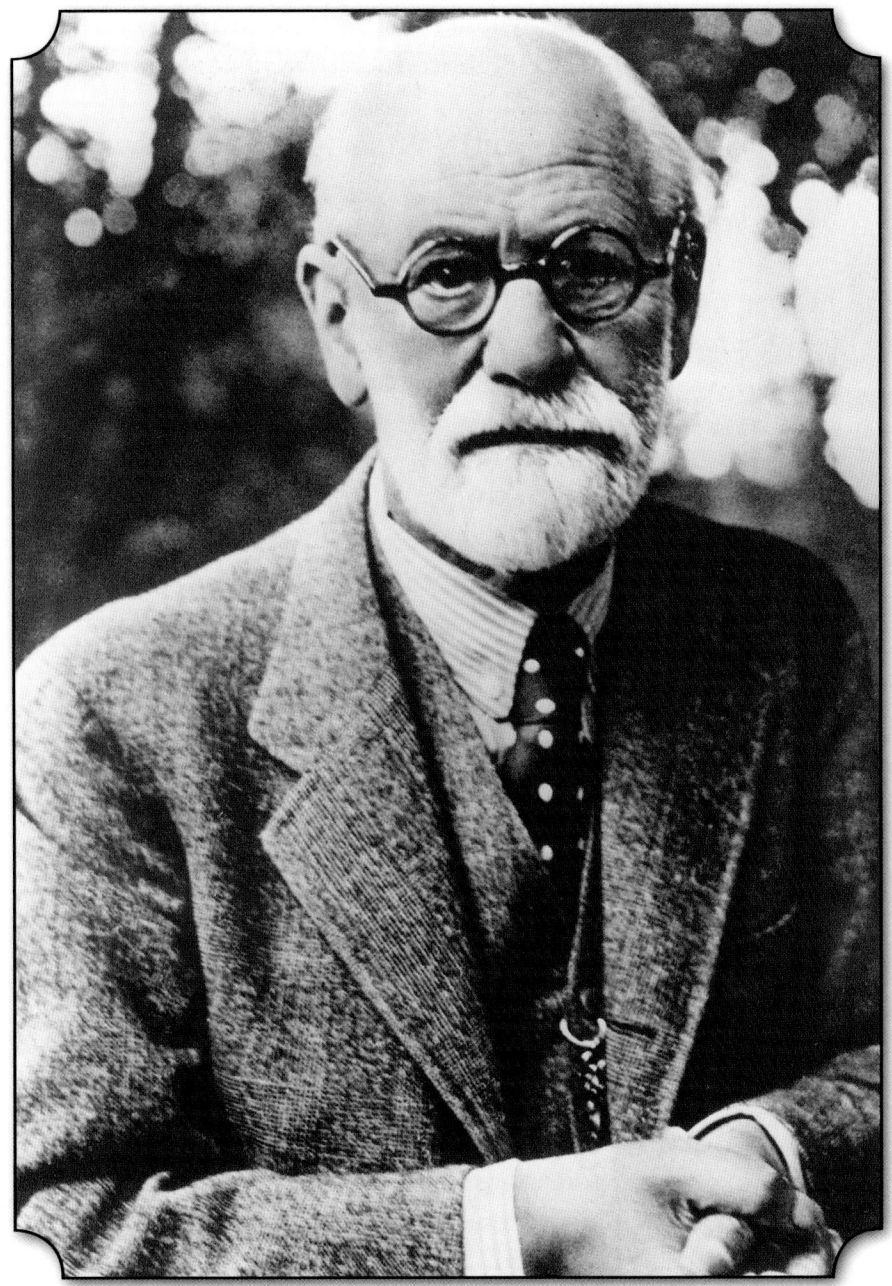

Psychoanalysis, or "depth psychology," became a highly influential method of treating mental disorders primarily because of the work of Sigmund Freud.

year his senior, who provided the model of intimate friend and hated rival that Freud reproduced often at later stages of his life.

In 1859 the Freud family was compelled for economic reasons to move to Leipzig and then a year after to Vienna, where Freud remained until the Nazi annexation of Austria 78 years later. Despite Freud's dislike of the imperial city, in part because of its citizens' frequent anti-Semitism, psychoanalysis reflected in significant ways the cultural and political context out of which it emerged. For example, Freud's sensitivity to the vulnerability of paternal authority within the psyche may well have been stimulated by the decline in power suffered by his father's generation, often liberal rationalists, in the Habsburg empire. So too his interest in the theme of the seduction of daughters was rooted in complicated ways in the context of Viennese attitudes toward female sexuality.

In 1873 Freud was graduated from the Sperl Gymnasium and, apparently inspired by a public reading of an essay by Goethe on nature, turned to medicine as a career. At the University of Vienna he worked with one of the leading physiologists of his day, Ernst von Brücke, an exponent of the materialist, antivitalist science of Hermann von Helmholtz. In 1882 he entered the General Hospital in Vienna as a clinical assistant to train with the psychiatrist Theodor Meynert and the professor of internal medicine Hermann Nothnagel. In 1885 Freud was appointed lecturer in neuropathology, having concluded important research on the brain's medulla. At this time he also developed an interest in the pharmaceutical benefits of cocaine, which he pursued for several years. Although some beneficial results were found in eye surgery, which have been credited to Freud's friend Carl Koller, the general outcome was disastrous. Not only did Freud's advocacy lead to a mortal addiction in another close friend, Ernst

Fleischl von Marxow, but it also tarnished his medical reputation for a time. Whether or not one interprets this episode in terms that call into question Freud's prudence as a scientist, it was of a piece with his lifelong willingness to attempt bold solutions to relieve human suffering.

Freud's scientific training remained of cardinal importance in his work, or at least in his own conception of it. In such writings as his "Entwurf einer Psychologie" (written 1895, published 1950; "Project for a Scientific Psychology") he affirmed his intention to find a physiological and materialist basis for his theories of the psyche. Here a mechanistic neurophysiological model vied with a more organismic, phylogenetic one in ways that demonstrate Freud's complicated debt to the science of his day.

In late 1885 Freud left Vienna to continue his studies of neuropathology at the Salpêtrière clinic in Paris, where he worked under the guidance of Jean-Martin Charcot. His 19 weeks in the French capital proved a turning point in his career, for Charcot's work with patients classified as "hysterics" introduced Freud to the possibility that psychological disorders might have their source in the mind rather than the brain. Charcot's demonstration of a link between hysterical symptoms, such as paralysis of a limb, and hypnotic suggestion implied the power of mental states rather than nerves in the etiology of disease. Although Freud was soon to abandon his faith in hypnosis, he returned to Vienna in February 1886 with the seed of his revolutionary psychological method implanted.

Several months after his return Freud married Martha Bernays, the daughter of a prominent Jewish family whose ancestors included a chief rabbi of Hamburg and Heinrich Heine. She was to bear six children, one of whom, Anna Freud, was to become a distinguished psychoanalyst in her own right. Although the glowing picture of their marriage painted by Ernest Jones in his biography of Freud has been nuanced by later scholars, it is clear that Martha Bernays Freud was a deeply sustaining presence during her husband's tumultuous career.

Shortly after his marriage Freud began his closest friendship, with the Berlin physician Wilhelm Fliess, whose role in the development of psychoanalysis has occasioned widespread debate. Throughout the 15 years of their intimacy Fliess provided Freud an invaluable interlocutor for his most daring ideas. Freud's belief in human bisexuality, his idea of erotogenic zones on the body, and perhaps even his imputation of sexuality to infants may well have been stimulated by their friendship.

A somewhat less controversial influence arose from the partnership Freud began with the physician Josef Breuer after his return from Paris. Freud turned to a clinical practice in neuropsychology, and the office he established at Berggasse 19 was to remain his consulting room for almost half a century. Before their collaboration began, during the early 1880s, Breuer had treated a patient named Bertha Pappenheim—or "Anna O.," as she became known in the literature—who was suffering from a variety of hysterical symptoms. Rather than using hypnotic suggestion, as had Charcot, Breuer allowed her to lapse into a state resembling autohypnosis, in which she would talk about the initial manifestations of her symptoms. To Breuer's surprise, the very act of verbalization seemed to provide some relief from their hold over her (although later scholarship has cast doubt on its permanence). "The talking cure" or "chimney sweeping," as Breuer and Anna O., respectively, called it, seemed to act cathartically to produce an abreaction, or discharge, of the pent-up emotional blockage at the root of the pathological behaviour.

Psychoanalytic Theory

Freud, still beholden to Charcot's hypnotic method, did not grasp the full implications of Breuer's experience until a decade later, when he developed the technique of free association. In part an extrapolation of the automatic writing promoted by the German Jewish writer Ludwig Börne a century before, in part a result of his own clinical experience with other hysterics, this revolutionary method was announced in the work Freud published jointly with Breuer in 1895, *Studien über Hysterie* (*Studies in Hysteria*). By encouraging the patient to express any random thoughts that came associatively to mind, the technique aimed at uncovering hitherto unarticulated material from the realm of the psyche that Freud, following a long tradition, called the unconscious. Because of its incompatibility with conscious thoughts or conflicts with other unconscious ones, this material was normally hidden, forgotten, or unavailable to conscious reflection. Difficulty in freely associating—sudden silences, stuttering, or the like—suggested to Freud the importance of the material struggling to be expressed, as well as the power of what he called the patient's defenses against that expression. Such blockages Freud dubbed resistance, which had to be broken down in order to reveal hidden conflicts. Unlike Charcot and Breuer, Freud came to the conclusion, based on his clinical experience with female hysterics, that the most insistent source of resisted material was sexual in nature. And even more momentously, he linked the etiology of neurotic symptoms to the same struggle between a sexual feeling or urge and the psychic defenses against it. Being able to bring that conflict to consciousness through free association and then probing its implications was thus a crucial step, he reasoned, on the road to relieving the symptom, which was best understood as an unwitting compromise formation between the wish and the defense.

Screen Memories

At first, however, Freud was uncertain about the precise status of the sexual component in this dynamic conception of the psyche. His patients seemed to recall actual experiences of early seductions, often incestuous in nature. Freud's initial impulse was to accept these as having happened. But then, as he disclosed in a now famous letter to Fliess of September 2, 1897, he concluded that, rather than being memories of actual events, these shocking recollections were the residues of infantile impulses and desires to be seduced by an adult. What was recalled was not a genuine memory but what he would later call a screen memory, or fantasy, hiding a primitive wish. That is, rather than stressing the corrupting initiative of adults in the etiology of neuroses, Freud concluded that the fantasies and yearnings of the child were at the root of later conflict.

The absolute centrality of his change of heart in the subsequent development of psychoanalysis cannot be doubted. For in attributing sexuality to children, emphasizing the causal power of fantasies, and establishing the importance of repressed desires, Freud laid the groundwork for what many have called the epic journey into his own psyche, which followed soon after the dissolution of his partnership with Breuer.

Freud's work on hysteria had focused on female sexuality and its potential for neurotic expression. To be fully universal, psychoanalysis—a term Freud coined in 1896—would also have to examine the male psyche in a condition of what might be called normality. It would have to become more than a psychotherapy and develop into a complete theory of the mind. To this end Freud accepted the enormous risk of generalizing from the experience he knew best: his own. Significantly, his self-analysis was both the first and the last in the history of the movement he spawned; all future analysts would have to undergo a training analysis with someone whose own analysis was ultimately traceable to Freud's of his disciples.

Freud's self-exploration was apparently enabled by a disturbing event in his life. In October 1896, Jakob Freud died shortly before his 81st birthday. Emotions were released in his son that he understood as having been long repressed, emotions concerning his earliest familial experiences and feelings. Beginning in earnest in July 1897, Freud attempted to reveal their meaning by drawing on a technique that had been available for millennia: the deciphering of dreams. Freud's contribution to the tradition of dream analysis was path-breaking, for in insisting on them as "the royal road to a knowledge of the unconscious," he provided a remarkably elaborate account of why dreams originate and how they function.

THE INTERPRETATION OF DREAMS

In what many commentators consider his master work, *Die Traumdeutung* (published in 1899, but given the date of the dawning century to emphasize its epochal character; *The Interpretation of Dreams*), he presented his findings. Interspersing evidence from his own dreams with evidence from those recounted in his clinical practice, Freud contended that dreams played a fundamental role in the psychic economy. The mind's energy—which Freud called libido and identified principally, but not exclusively, with the sexual drive—was a fluid and malleable force capable of excessive and disturbing power. Needing to be discharged to ensure pleasure and prevent pain, it sought whatever outlet it might find. If denied the gratification provided by direct motor action, libidinal energy could seek its release through mental channels. Or, in the language of *The Interpretation of Dreams*, a wish can be satisfied by an imaginary wish fulfillment. All dreams, Freud claimed, even nightmares manifesting apparent anxiety, are the fulfillment of such wishes.

More precisely, dreams are the disguised expression of wish fulfillments. Like neurotic symptoms, they are the effects of compromises in the psyche between desires and prohibitions in conflict with their realization. Although sleep can relax the power of the mind's diurnal censorship of forbidden desires, such censorship, nonetheless, persists in part during nocturnal existence. Dreams, therefore, have to be decoded to be understood, and not merely because they are actually forbidden desires experienced in distorted fashion. For dreams undergo further revision in the process of being recounted to the analyst.

The Interpretation of Dreams provides a hermeneutic for the unmasking of the dream's disguise, or dreamwork, as Freud called it. The manifest content of the dream, that which is remembered and reported, must be understood as veiling a latent meaning. Dreams defy logical entailment and narrative coherence, for they intermingle the residues of immediate daily experience with the deepest, often most infantile wishes. Yet they can be ultimately decoded by attending to four basic activities of the dreamwork and reversing their mystifying effect.

The first of these activities, condensation, operates through the fusion of several different elements into one. As such, it exemplifies one of the key operations of psychic life, which Freud called overdetermination. No direct correspondence between a simple manifest content and its multidimensional latent counterpart can be assumed. The second activity of the dreamwork, displacement, refers to the decentring of dream thoughts, so that the most urgent wish is often obliquely or marginally represented on the manifest level. Displacement also means the associative substitution of one signifier in the dream for another, say, the king for one's father. The third activity Freud called representation, by which he meant the transformation of thoughts into images. Decoding a dream thus means translating such visual representations back into intersubjectively available language through free association. The final function of the dreamwork is secondary revision, which provides some order and intelligibility to the dream by supplementing its content with narrative coherence. The process of dream interpretation thus reverses the direction of the dreamwork, moving from the level of the conscious recounting of the dream through the preconscious back beyond censorship into the unconscious itself.

FURTHER THEORETICAL DEVELOPMENT

In 1904 Freud published *Zur Psychopathologie des Alltagslebens* (*The Psychopathology of Everyday Life*), in which he explored such seemingly insignificant errors as slips of the tongue or pen (later colloquially called Freudian slips), misreadings, or forgetting of names. These errors Freud understood to have symptomatic and thus interpretable importance. But unlike dreams they need not betray a repressed infantile wish yet can arise from more immediate hostile, jealous, or egoistic causes.

In 1905 Freud extended the scope of this analysis by examining *Der Witz und seine Beziehung zum Unbewussten* (*Jokes and Their Relation to the Unconscious*). Invoking the idea of "joke-work" as a process comparable to dreamwork, he also acknowledged the double-sided quality of jokes, at once consciously contrived and unconsciously revealing. Seemingly innocent phenomena like puns or jests are as open to interpretation as more obviously tendentious, obscene, or hostile jokes. The explosive response often produced by successful humour, Freud contended, owes its power to the orgasmic release of unconscious impulses, aggressive as well as sexual. But insofar as jokes are more deliberate than dreams or slips, they draw on the rational dimension of the psyche that Freud was to call the ego as much as on what he was to call the id.

In 1905 Freud also published the work that first thrust him into the limelight as the alleged champion of a pansexualist understanding of the mind: *Drei Abhandlungen zur Sexualtheorie* (*Three Contributions to the Sexual Theory*, later translated as *Three Essays on the Theory of Sexuality*), revised and expanded in subsequent editions. The work established Freud, along with Richard von Kraft-Ebing, Havelock Ellis, Albert Moll, and Iwan Bloch, as a pioneer in the serious study of sexology. Here he outlined in greater detail than before his reasons for emphasizing the sexual component in the development of both normal and pathological behaviour. Although not as reductionist as popularly assumed, Freud nonetheless extended the concept of sexuality beyond conventional usage to include a panoply of erotic impulses from the earliest childhood years on. Distinguishing between sexual aims (the act toward which instincts strive) and sexual objects (the person, organ, or physical entity eliciting attraction), he elaborated a repertoire of sexually generated behaviour of astonishing variety. Beginning very early in life, imperiously insistent on its gratification, remarkably plastic in its expression, and open to easy maldevelopment, sexuality, Freud concluded, is the prime mover in a great deal of human behaviour.

SEXUALITY AND DEVELOPMENT

To spell out the formative development of the sexual drive, Freud focused on the progressive replacement of erotogenic zones in the body by others. An originally polymorphous sexuality first seeks gratification orally through sucking at the mother's breast, an object for which other surrogates can later be provided. Initially unable to distinguish between self and breast, the infant soon comes to appreciate its mother as the first external love object. Later Freud would contend that even before that moment, the child can treat its own body as such an object, going beyond undifferentiated autoeroticism to a narcissistic love for the self as such. After the oral phase, during the second year, the child's erotic focus shifts to its anus, stimulated by the struggle over toilet training. During the anal phase the child's pleasure in defecation is confronted with the demands of self-control. The third phase, lasting from about the fourth to the sixth year, he called the phallic. Because Freud relied on male sexuality as the norm of development, his analysis of this phase aroused considerable opposition, especially because he claimed its major concern is castration anxiety.

To grasp what Freud meant by this fear, it is necessary to understand one of his central contentions. As has been stated, the death of Freud's father was the trauma that permitted him to delve into his own psyche. Not only did Freud experience the expected grief, but he also expressed disappointment, resentment, and even hostility toward his father in the dreams he analyzed at the time. In the process of abandoning the seduction theory he recognized the source of the anger as his own psyche rather than anything objectively done by his father. Turning, as he often did, to evidence from literary and mythical texts as anticipations of his psychological insights, Freud interpreted that source in terms of Sophocles' tragedy *Oedipus Rex*. The universal applicability of its plot, he conjectured, lies in the desire of every male child to sleep with his mother and remove the obstacle to the realization of that wish, his father. What he later dubbed the Oedipus complex presents the child with a critical problem, for the unrealizable yearning at its root provokes an imagined response on the part of the father: the threat of castration.

The phallic stage can only be successfully surmounted if the Oedipus complex with its accompanying castration anxiety can be resolved. According to Freud, this resolution can occur if the boy finally suppresses his sexual desire for the mother, entering a period of so-called latency, and internalizes the reproachful prohibition of the father, making it his own with the construction of that part of the psyche Freud called the superego or the conscience.

The blatantly phallocentric bias of this account, which was supplemented by a highly controversial assumption of penis envy in the already castrated female child, proved troublesome for subsequent psychoanalytic theory. Not surprisingly, later analysts of female sexuality have paid more attention to the girl's relations with the pre-Oedipal mother than to the vicissitudes of the Oedipus complex. Anthropological challenges to the universality of the complex have also been damaging, although it has been possible to redescribe it in terms that lift it out of the specific familial dynamics of Freud's own day. If the creation of culture is understood as the institution of kinship structures based on exogamy, then the Oedipal drama reflects the deeper struggle between natural desire and cultural authority.

Freud, however, always maintained the intrapsychic importance of the Oedipus complex, whose successful resolution is the precondition for the transition through latency to the mature sexuality he called the genital phase. Here the parent of the opposite sex is conclusively abandoned in favour of a more suitable love object able to reciprocate reproductively useful passion. In the case of the girl, disappointment over the nonexistence of a penis is transcended by the rejection of her mother in favour of a father figure instead. In both cases, sexual maturity means heterosexual, procreatively inclined, genitally focused behaviour.

Sexual development, however, is prone to troubling maladjustments preventing this outcome if the various stages are unsuccessfully negotiated. Fixation of sexual aims or objects can occur at any particular moment, caused either by an actual trauma or the blockage of a powerful libidinal urge. If the fixation is allowed to express itself directly at a later age, the result is what was then generally called a perversion. If, however, some part of the psyche prohibits such overt expression, then, Freud contended, the repressed and censored impulse produces neurotic symptoms, neuroses being conceptualized as the negative of perversions. Neurotics repeat the desired act in repressed form, without conscious memory of its origin or the ability to confront and work it through in the present.

In addition to the neurosis of hysteria, with its conversion of affective conflicts into bodily symptoms, Freud developed complicated etiological explanations for other typical neurotic behaviour, such as obsessive-compulsions, paranoia, and narcissism. These he called psychoneuroses, because of their rootedness in childhood conflicts, as opposed to the actual neuroses such as hypochondria, neurasthenia, and anxiety neurosis, which are due to problems in the present (the last, for example, being caused by the physical suppression of sexual release).

Freud's elaboration of his therapeutic technique during these years focused on the implications of a specific element in the relationship between patient and analyst, an element whose power he first began to recognize in reflecting on Breuer's work with Anna O. Although later scholarship has cast doubt on its veracity, Freud's account of the episode was as follows. An intense rapport between Breuer and his patient had taken an alarming turn when Anna divulged her strong sexual desire for him. Breuer, who recognized the stirrings of reciprocal feelings, broke off his treatment out of an understandable confusion about the ethical implications of acting on these impulses. Freud came to see in this troubling interaction the effects of a more pervasive phenomenon, which he called transference (or in the case of the analyst's desire for the patient, counter-transference). Produced by the projection of feelings, transference, he reasoned, is the reenactment of childhood urges cathected (invested) on a new object. As such, it is the essential tool in the analytic cure, for by bringing to the surface repressed emotions and allowing them to be examined in a clinical setting, transference can permit their being worked through in the present. That is, affective remembrance can be the antidote to neurotic repetition.

It was largely to facilitate transference that Freud developed his celebrated technique of having the patient lie on a couch, not looking directly at the analyst, and free to fantasize with as little intrusion of the analyst's real personality as possible. Restrained and neutral, the analyst functions as a screen for the displacement of early emotions, both erotic and aggressive. Transference onto the analyst is itself a kind of neurosis, but one in the service of an ultimate working through of the conflicting feelings it expresses. Only certain illnesses, however, are open to this treatment, for it demands the ability to redirect libidinal energy outward. The psychoses, Freud sadly concluded, are based on the redirection of libido back onto the patient's ego and cannot therefore be relieved by transference in the analytic situation. How successful psychoanalytic therapy has been in the treatment of psychoneuroses remains, however, a matter of considerable dispute.

Although Freud's theories were offensive to many in the Vienna of his day, they began to attract a cosmopolitan group of supporters in the early 1900s. In 1902 the Psychological Wednesday Circle began to gather in Freud's waiting room with a number of future luminaries in the psychoanalytic movements in attendance. Alfred Adler and Wilhelm Stekel were often joined by guests such as Sándor Ferenczi, Carl Gustav Jung, Otto Rank, Ernest Jones, Max Eitingon, and A.A. Brill. In 1908 the group was renamed the Vienna Psychoanalytic Society and held its first international congress in Salzburg. In the same year the first branch society was opened in Berlin. In 1909 Freud, along with Jung and Ferenczi, made a historic trip to Clark University in Worcester, Mass. The lectures he gave there were soon published as *Über Psychoanalyse* (1910; *The Origin and Development of Psychoanalysis*), the first of several introductions he wrote for a general audience. Along with a series of vivid case studies—the most famous known colloquially as "Dora" (1905), "Little Hans" (1909), "The Rat Man" (1909), "The Psychotic Dr. Schreber" (1911), and "The Wolf Man" (1918)—they made his ideas known to a wider public.

As might be expected of a movement whose treatment emphasized the power of transference and the ubiquity of Oedipal conflict, its early history is a tale rife with dissension, betrayal, apostasy, and excommunication. The most widely noted schisms occurred with Adler in 1911, Stekel in 1912, and Jung in 1913; these were followed by later breaks with Ferenczi, Rank, and Wilhelm Reich in the 1920s. Despite efforts by loyal disciples like Ernest Jones to exculpate Freud from blame, subsequent research concerning his relations with former disciples like Viktor Tausk have clouded the picture considerably. Critics of the hagiographic legend of Freud have, in fact, had a relatively easy time documenting the tension between

Freud's aspirations to scientific objectivity and the extraordinarily fraught personal context in which his ideas were developed and disseminated. Even well after Freud's death, his archivists' insistence on limiting access to potentially embarrassing material in his papers has reinforced the impression that the psychoanalytic movement resembled more a sectarian church than a scientific community (at least as the latter is ideally understood).

Toward a General Theory

If the troubled history of its institutionalization served to call psychoanalysis into question in certain quarters, so too did its founder's penchant for extrapolating his clinical findings into a more ambitious general theory. As he admitted to Fliess in 1900, "I am actually not a man of science at all.... I am nothing but a conquistador by temperament, an adventurer." Freud's so-called metapsychology soon became the basis for wide-ranging speculations about cultural, social, artistic, religious, and anthropological phenomena. Composed of a complicated and often revised mixture of economic, dynamic, and topographical elements, the metapsychology was developed in a series of 12 papers Freud composed during World War I, only some of which were published in his lifetime. Their general findings appeared in two books in the 1920s: *Jenseits des Lustprinzips* (1920; *Beyond the Pleasure Principle*) and *Das Ich und das Es* (1923; *The Ego and the Id*).

In these works, Freud attempted to clarify the relationship between his earlier topographical division of the psyche into the unconscious, preconscious, and conscious and his subsequent structural categorization into id, ego, and superego. The id was defined in terms of the most primitive urges for gratification in the infant, urges dominated by the desire for pleasure through the release of tension and the cathexis of energy. Ruled by no laws of logic, indifferent to the demands of expediency, unconstrained by the resistance of external reality, the id is ruled by what Freud called the primary process directly expressing somatically generated instincts. Through the inevitable experience of frustration the infant learns to adapt itself to the exigencies of reality. The secondary process that results leads to the growth of the ego, which follows what Freud called the reality principle in contradistinction to the pleasure principle dominating the id. Here the need to delay gratification in the service of self-preservation is slowly learned in an effort to thwart the anxiety produced by unfulfilled desires. What Freud termed defense mechanisms are developed by the ego to deal with such conflicts. Repression is the most fundamental, but Freud also posited an entire repertoire of others, including reaction formation, isolation, undoing, denial, displacement, and rationalization.

The last component in Freud's trichotomy, the superego, develops from the internalization of society's moral commands through identification with parental dictates during the resolution of the Oedipus complex. Only partly conscious, the superego gains some of its punishing force by borrowing certain aggressive elements in the id, which are turned inward against the ego and produce feelings of guilt. But it is largely through the internalization of social norms that the superego is constituted, an acknowledgement that prevents psychoanalysis from conceptualizing the psyche in purely biologistic or individualistic terms.

Freud's understanding of the primary process underwent a crucial shift in the course of his career. Initially he counterposed a libidinal drive that seeks sexual pleasure to a self-preservation drive whose telos is survival. But in 1914, while examining the phenomenon of narcissism, he came to consider the latter instinct as merely a variant of the former. Unable to accept so monistic a drive theory,

Freud sought a new dualistic alternative. He arrived at the speculative assertion that there exists in the psyche an innate, regressive drive for stasis that aims to end life's inevitable tension. This striving for rest he christened the Nirvana principle and the drive underlying it the death instinct, or Thanatos, which he could substitute for self-preservation as the contrary of the life instinct, or Eros.

SOCIAL AND CULTURAL STUDIES

Freud's mature instinct theory is in many ways a metaphysical construct, comparable to Bergson's *élan vital* or Schopenhauer's Will. Emboldened by its formulation, Freud launched a series of audacious studies that took him well beyond his clinician's consulting room. These he had already commenced with investigations of Leonardo da Vinci (1910) and the novel *Gradiva* by Wilhelm Jensen (1907). Here Freud attempted to psychoanalyze works of art as symbolic expressions of their creator's psychodynamics.

The fundamental premise that permitted Freud to examine cultural phenomena was called sublimation in the *Three Essays*. The appreciation or creation of ideal beauty, Freud contended, is rooted in primitive sexual urges that are transfigured in culturally elevating ways. Unlike repression, which produces only neurotic symptoms whose meaning is unknown even to the sufferer, sublimation is a conflict-free resolution of repression, which leads to intersubjectively available cultural works. Although potentially reductive in its implications, the psychoanalytic interpretation of culture can be justly called one of the most powerful "hermeneutics of suspicion," to borrow the French philosopher Paul Ricoeur's phrase, because it debunks idealist notions of high culture as the alleged transcendence of baser concerns.

Freud extended the scope of his theories to include anthropological and social psychological speculation as well in *Totem und Tabu* (1913; *Totem and Taboo*). Drawing on Sir James Frazer's explorations of the Australian Aborigines, he interpreted the mixture of fear and reverence for the totemic animal in terms of the child's attitude toward the parent of the same sex. The Aborigines' insistence on exogamy was a complicated defense against the strong incestuous desires felt by the child for the parent of the opposite sex. Their religion was thus a phylogenetic anticipation of the ontogenetic Oedipal drama played out in modern man's psychic development. But whereas the latter was purely an intrapsychic phenomenon based on fantasies and fears, the former, Freud boldly suggested, was based on actual historical events. Freud speculated that the rebellion of sons against dominating fathers for control over women had culminated in actual parricide. Ultimately producing remorse, this violent act led to atonement through incest taboos and the prohibitions against harming the father-substitute, the totemic object or animal. When the fraternal clan replaced the patriarchal horde, true society emerged. For renunciation of individual aspirations to replace the slain father and a shared sense of guilt in the primal crime led to a contractual agreement to end internecine struggle and band together instead. The totemic ancestor then could evolve into the more impersonal God of the great religions.

A subsequent effort to explain social solidarity, *Massenpsychologie und Ich-analyse* (1921; *Group Psychology and the Analysis of the Ego*), drew on the antidemocratic crowd psychologists of the late 19th century, most notably Gustave Le Bon. Here the disillusionment with liberal, rational politics that some have seen as the seedbed of much of Freud's work was at its most explicit (the only competitor being the debunking psychobiography of

Woodrow Wilson he wrote jointly with William Bullitt in 1930, which was not published until 1967). All mass phenomena, Freud suggested, are characterized by intensely regressive emotional ties stripping individuals of their self-control and independence. Rejecting possible alternative explanations such as hypnotic suggestion or imitation and unwilling to follow Jung in postulating a group mind, Freud emphasized instead individual libidinal ties to the group's leader. Group formation is like regression to a primal horde with the leader as the original father. Drawing on the army and the Roman Catholic Church as his examples, Freud never seriously considered less authoritarian modes of collective behaviour.

Religion, Civilization, and Discontents

Freud's bleak appraisal of social and political solidarity was replicated, if in somewhat more nuanced form, in his attitude toward religion. Although many accounts of Freud's development have discerned debts to one or another aspect of his Jewish background, debts Freud himself partly acknowledged, his avowed position was deeply irreligious. As noted in the account of *Totem and Taboo*, he always attributed the belief in divinities ultimately to the displaced worship of human ancestors. One of the most potent sources of his break with former disciples like Jung was precisely this skepticism toward spirituality.

In his 1907 essay "Zwangshandlungen und Religionsübungen" ("Obsessive Acts and Religious Practices," later translated as "Obsessive Actions and Religious Practices") Freud had already contended that obsessional neuroses are private religious systems and religions themselves no more than the obsessional neuroses of mankind. Twenty years later, in *Die Zukunft einer Illusion* (1927; *The Future of an Illusion*), he elaborated this argument, adding that belief in God is a mythic reproduction of the universal state of infantile helplessness. Like an idealized father, God is the projection of childish wishes for an omnipotent protector. If children can outgrow their dependence, he concluded with cautious optimism, then humanity may also hope to leave behind its immature heteronomy.

The simple Enlightenment faith underlying this analysis quickly elicited critical comment, which led to its modification. In an exchange of letters with the French novelist Romain Rolland, Freud came to acknowledge a more intractable source of religious sentiment. The opening section of his next speculative tract, *Das Unbehagen in der Kultur* (1930; *Civilization and Its Discontents*), was devoted to what Rolland had dubbed the oceanic feeling. Freud described it as a sense of indissoluble oneness with the universe, which mystics in particular have celebrated as the fundamental religious experience. Its origin, Freud claimed, is nostalgia for the pre-Oedipal infant's sense of unity with its mother. Although still rooted in infantile helplessness, religion thus derives to some extent from the earliest stage of postnatal development. Regressive longings for its restoration are possibly stronger than those for a powerful father and thus cannot be worked through by way of a collective resolution of the Oedipus complex.

Civilization and Its Discontents, written after the onset of Freud's struggle with cancer of the jaw and in the midst of the rise of European Fascism, was a profoundly unconsoling book. Focusing on the prevalence of human guilt and the impossibility of achieving unalloyed happiness, Freud contended that no social solution of the discontents of mankind is possible. All civilizations, no matter how well planned, can provide only partial relief. For aggression among men is not due to unequal property relations or political injustice, which can be rectified by laws, but rather to the death instinct redirected outward.

Even Eros, Freud suggested, is not fully in harmony with civilization, for the libidinal ties creating collective solidarity are aim-inhibited and diffuse rather than directly sexual. Thus, there is likely to be tension between the urge for sexual gratification and the sublimated love for mankind. Furthermore, because Eros and Thanatos are themselves at odds, conflict and the guilt it engenders are virtually inevitable. The best to be hoped for is a life in which the repressive burdens of civilization are in rough balance with the realization of instinctual gratification and the sublimated love for mankind. But reconciliation of nature and culture is impossible, for the price of any civilization is the guilt produced by the necessary thwarting of man's instinctual drives. Although elsewhere Freud had postulated mature, heterosexual genitality and the capacity to work productively as the hallmarks of health and urged that "where id is, there shall ego be," it is clear that he held out no hope for any collective relief from the discontents of civilization. He only offered an ethic of resigned authenticity, which taught the wisdom of living without the possibility of redemption, either religious or secular.

Last Days

Freud's final major work, *Der Mann Moses und die monotheistische Religion* (1938; *Moses and Monotheism*), was more than just the "historical novel" he had initially thought to subtitle it. Moses had long been a figure of capital importance for Freud; indeed Michelangelo's famous statue of Moses had been the subject of an essay written in 1914. The book itself sought to solve the mystery of Moses' origins by claiming that he was actually an aristocratic Egyptian by birth who had chosen the Jewish people to keep alive an earlier monotheistic religion. Too stern and demanding a taskmaster, Moses was slain in a Jewish revolt, and a second, more pliant leader, also called Moses, rose in his place. The guilt engendered by the parricidal act was, however, too much to endure, and the Jews ultimately returned to the religion given them by the original Moses as the two figures were merged into one in their memories. Here Freud's ambivalence about his religious roots and his father's authority was allowed to pervade a highly fanciful story that reveals more about its author than its ostensible subject.

Moses and Monotheism was published in the year Hitler invaded Austria. Freud was forced to flee to England. His books were among the first to be burned, as the fruits of a "Jewish science," when the Nazis took over Germany. Although psychotherapy was not banned in the Third Reich, where Field Marshall Hermann Göring's cousin headed an official institute, psychoanalysis essentially went into exile, most notably to North America and England. Freud himself died only a few weeks after World War II broke out, at a time when his worst fears about the irrationality lurking behind the facade of civilization were being realized. Freud's death did not, however, hinder the reception and dissemination of his ideas. A plethora of Freudian schools emerged to develop psychoanalysis in different directions. In fact, despite the relentless and often compelling challenges mounted against virtually all of his ideas, Freud has remained one of the most potent figures in the intellectual landscape of the 20th century.

DANIEL HALE WILLIAMS
(born Jan. 18, 1858, Hollidaysburg, Pa., U.S.–died Aug. 4, 1931, Idlewild, Mich.)

Daniel Hale Williams was an American physician and founder of Provident Hospital in Chicago, credited with the first successful heart surgery.

Williams graduated from Chicago Medical College in 1883. He served as surgeon for the South Side Dispensary (1884–92) and physician for the Protestant Orphan Asylum (1884–93). In response to the lack of opportunity for blacks in the medical professions, he founded (1891) the nation's first interracial hospital, Provident, to provide training for black interns and the first school for black nurses in the United States. He was a surgeon at Provident (1892–93, 1898–1912) and surgeon in chief of Freedmen's Hospital, Washington, D.C. (1894–98), where he established another school for black nurses.

It was at Provident Hospital that Williams performed daring heart surgery on July 10, 1893. Although contemporary medical opinion disapproved of surgical treatment of heart wounds, Williams opened the patient's thoracic cavity without aid of blood transfusions or modern anesthetics and antibiotics. During the surgery he examined the heart, sutured a wound of the pericardium (the sac surrounding the heart), and closed the chest. The patient lived at least 20 years following the surgery. Williams' procedure is cited as the first recorded repair of the pericardium; some sources, however, cite a similar operation performed by H.C. Dalton of St. Louis in 1891.

Williams later served on the staffs of Cook County Hospital (1903–09) and St. Luke's Hospital (1912–31), both in Chicago. From 1899 he was professor of clinical surgery at Meharry Medical College in Nashville, Tenn., and was a member of the Illinois State Board of Health (1889–91). He published several articles on surgery in medical journals. Williams became the only black charter member of the American College of Surgeons in 1913.

REBECCA LEE DORSEY

(born Aug. 30, 1859, Md., U.S.–died March 29, 1954, Los Angeles, Calif.)

Rebecca Lee Dorsey was a U.S. physician who was a pioneer in the field of endocrinology and the study of hormones. She was one of the first female doctors to practice medicine in Los Angeles. According to her unpublished memoirs (which are thought to contain significant embellishments), Dorsey was self-sufficient from age nine; she nursed her mother through tuberculosis and worked to earn money for her siblings' care. She later moved from her childhood home in Maryland to Philadelphia and became a servant, using the money to put herself through grammar school. She attended Wellesley College and supported herself by doing menial jobs for other students. Similarly, while earning her medical degree at Boston University, she cared for sick people in order to provide herself with an income. During that time she developed symptoms of tuberculosis. She graduated in June 1882 and the following year traveled to Europe, where she spent the next few years studying and pursuing treatment for her illness. Dorsey underwent an experimental treatment for the disease, and her health improved. After returning to the United States, she settled in Los Angeles in 1886.

Dorsey began her own medical practice and worked out of St. Vincent's Medical Center. She drove a horse and buggy to the various homes and ranches that required her services. Her practice concentrated on obstetrics, pediatrics, and, later, endocrinology, and she was said to have been the attending physician at over 4,000 births during her lifetime. Perhaps her most famous delivery was Earl Warren, who grew up to become a governor of California and chief justice of the U.S. Supreme Court. Dorsey said that she never lost a baby or mother during delivery and attributed that accomplishment to her adherance to four rules: (1) she had a perfect understanding of the measurement of a mother's pelvis as well as the size and weight of the child; (2) she advocated good prenatal care; (3) she had a strictly aseptic technique; and (4) she made sure that the afterbirth was completely delivered. She also claimed that she never had a single case of puerperal, or childbed, fever among her patients, owing to her knowledge of sterilization, which she learned from Joseph Lister during her time in Europe. Dorsey was also skilled in the use of forceps and caused no serious injury to any of the babies she delivered.

Dorsey claimed to have performed the first three successful appendectomies in Los Angeles county and to have administered the first diphtheria inoculation in Los Angeles about 1893. She also helped establish the first training school for nurses in the city. During World War I she consulted for the U.S. secretary of war regarding the number of women nurses available in the United States and offered suggestions for a rapid multiplication of trained women available in a time of emergency. After 60 years of practice, she retired to her ranch near Indio, Calif., in the Coachella Valley, where she became a pioneer in date farming.

WILLIAM BATESON

(born Aug. 8, 1861, Whitby, Yorkshire, England–died Feb. 8, 1926, London)

William Bateson was a biologist who founded and named the science of genetics and whose experiments provided evidence basic to the modern understanding of heredity. A dedicated evolutionist, he cited embryo studies to support his contention in 1885 that chordates evolved from primitive echinoderms, a view now widely accepted. In 1894 he published his conclusion (*Materials for the Study of Variation*) that evolution could not occur through a continuous variation of species, since distinct features often appeared or disappeared suddenly in plants and animals. Realizing that discontinuous variation could be understood only after something was known about the inheritance of traits, Bateson began work on the experimental breeding of plants and animals.

In 1900, he discovered an article, "Experiments with Plant Hybrids," written by Gregor Mendel, an Austrian monk, 34 years earlier. The paper, found in the same year by Hugo de Vries, Carl Correns, and Erich Tschermak von Seysenegg, dealt with the appearance of certain features in successive generations of garden peas. Bateson noted that his breeding results were explained perfectly by Mendel's paper and that the monk had succinctly described the transmission of elements governing heritable traits in his plants.

Bateson translated Mendel's paper into English and during the next 10 years became Mendel's champion in England, corroborating his principles experimentally. He published, with Reginald Punnett, the results of a series of breeding experiments (1905–08) that not only extended Mendel's principles to animals (poultry) but showed also that certain features were consistently inherited together, apparently counter to Mendel's findings. This phenomenon, which came to be termed linkage, is now known to be the result of the occurrence of genes located in close proximity on the same chromosome. Bateson's experiments also demonstrated a dependence of certain characters on two or more genes. Unfortunately, he misinterpreted his results, refusing to accept the interpretation of linkage advanced by the geneticist Thomas Hunt Morgan. In fact, he opposed Morgan's entire chromosome theory, advocating his own vibratory theory of inheritance, founded on laws of force and motion, a concept that found little acceptance among other scientists.

Bateson became, at the University of Cambridge, the first British professor of genetics (1908). He left this chair in 1910 to spend the rest of his life directing the John Innes Horticultural Institution at Merton, South London (later moved to Norwich), transforming it into a centre for genetic research. His books include *Mendel's Principles of Heredity* (1902, 2nd edition published in 1909) and *Problems of Genetics* (1913).

ABRAHAM FLEXNER

(born Nov. 13, 1866, Louisville, Ky., U.S.–died Sept. 21, 1959, Falls Church, Va.)

Abraham Flexner was an educator who played a major role in the introduction of modern medical and science education to American colleges and universities.

Founder and director of a progressive college-preparatory school in Louisville (1890–1904), Flexner issued an appraisal of American educational institutions (*The American College: A Criticism;* 1908) that earned him a Carnegie Foundation commission to survey the quality of the 155 medical colleges in the United States and Canada. His report (1910) had an immediate and sensational impact on American medical education. Many of the colleges that were severely criticized by Flexner closed soon after publication of the report; others initiated extensive revisions of their policies and curricula.

In the report, Flexner pointed out that medical education actually is a form of education rather than a mysterious process of professional initiation or apprenticeship. As such, it needs an academic staff, working full-time in their departments, whose whole responsibility is to their professed subject and to the students studying it. Medical education, the report further stated, needs laboratories, libraries, teaching rooms, and ready access to a large hospital, the administration of which should reflect the presence and influence of the academic staff. Thus the nature of the teaching hospital was also influenced.

As secretary to the Rockefeller Foundation's General Education Board (1913–28), he actively channeled more than half a billion dollars from private donors into the improvement of American medical education from 1913 to 1929 in such matters as were stressed in the Flexner report. In 1930 he realized his ambition to create a model centre for higher learning when he founded the Institute for Advanced Study, Princeton, N.J. As the institute's first director (1930–39), Flexner gathered together several of the world's most distinguished scientists, highlighted by the arrival there in 1933 of Albert Einstein.

KARL LANDSTEINER

(born June 14, 1868, Vienna, Austrian Empire [Austria]–died June 26, 1943, New York, N.Y., U.S.)

Karl Landsteiner was an Austrian American immunologist and pathologist who received the 1930 Nobel Prize for Physiology or Medicine for his discovery of the major blood groups and the development of the ABO system of blood typing that has made blood transfusion a routine medical practice.

After receiving his M.D. in 1891 from the University of Vienna, Landsteiner studied organic chemistry with many notable scientists in Europe, including the German chemist Emil Fischer. In 1897 he returned to the University of

Vienna, where he pursued his interest in the emerging field of immunology and in 1901 published his discovery of the human ABO blood group system. At that time, although it was known that the mixing of blood from two individuals could result in clumping, or agglutination, of red blood cells, the underlying mechanism of this phenomenon was not understood. Landsteiner discovered the cause of agglutination to be an immunological reaction that occurs when antibodies are produced by the host against donated blood cells. This immune response is elicited because blood from different individuals may vary with respect to certain antigens located on the surface of red blood cells. Landsteiner identified three such antigens, which he labeled A, B, and C (later changed to O). A fourth blood type, later named AB, was identified the following year. He found that if a person with one blood type—A, for example—receives blood from an individual of a different blood type, such as B, the host's immune system will not recognize the B antigens on the donor blood cells and thus will consider them to be foreign and dangerous, as it would regard an infectious microorganism. To defend the body from this perceived threat, the host's immune system will produce antibodies against the B antigens, and agglutination will occur as the antibodies bind to the B antigens. Landsteiner's work made it possible to determine blood type and thus paved the way for blood transfusions to be carried out safely. Landsteiner also discovered other blood factors during his career: the M, N, and P factors, which he identified in 1927 with Philip Levine, and the Rhesus (Rh) system, in 1940 with Alexander Wiener.

In addition to his study of human blood groups, Landsteiner made a number of other important contributions to science. He and the Romanian bacteriologist Constantin Levaditi discovered that a microorganism is responsible for poliomyelitis and laid the groundwork for the development of the polio vaccine. Landsteiner also helped identify the microorganisms responsible for syphilis. However, he considered his greatest work to be his investigations into antigen-antibody interactions, which he carried out primarily at Rockefeller Institute (now called Rockefeller University) in New York City (1922–43). In this research Landsteiner used small organic molecules called haptens—which stimulate antibody production only when combined with a larger molecule, such as protein—to demonstrate how small variations in a molecule's structure can cause great changes in antibody production. Landsteiner summarized his work in *The Specificity of Serological Reactions* (1936), a classic text that helped establish the field of immunochemistry.

FLORENCE RENA SABIN

(born Nov. 9, 1871, Central City, Colo., U.S.–died Oct. 3, 1953, Denver, Colo.)

Florence Rena Sabin was an American anatomist and investigator of the lymphatic system who was considered to be one of the leading women scientists of the United States.

Sabin was educated in Denver, Colo., and in Vermont and she graduated from Smith College in Massachusetts, in 1893. After teaching in Denver and at Smith to earn tuition money, she entered the Johns Hopkins University Medical School in Baltimore, Md., in 1896. While a student she demonstrated a particular gift for laboratory work; her model of the brain stem of a newborn infant was widely reproduced for use as a teaching model in medical schools. After graduation in 1900 she interned at Johns Hopkins Hospital for a year and then returned to the medical school to conduct research under a fellowship awarded by the Baltimore Association for the Advancement of University Education of Women. In 1901 she published *An Atlas of the Medulla and Midbrain*, which became a popular medical text. In 1902, when Johns Hopkins finally abandoned its policy of not appointing women to its medical faculty, Sabin was named an assistant in anatomy, and she became in 1917 the school's first female full professor.

For a number of years Sabin's research centred on the lymphatic system, and her demonstration that lymphatic vessels develop from a special layer of cells in certain fetal veins, rather than, as prevailing theory held, from intercellular spaces, established her as a researcher of the first rank. She then turned to the study of blood, blood vessels, and blood cells and made numerous discoveries regarding their origin and development. In 1924 she was elected president of the American Association of Anatomists, and in 1925 she was elected to the National Academy of Sciences; in both cases she was the first woman to be so honoured.

Also in 1925 she accepted an invitation to join the Rockefeller Institute for Medical Research (now Rockefeller University), where she was also the first woman member. There she conducted research on tuberculosis, particularly the role of monocytes in forming tubercles. In 1934 she published a biography of her early mentor at Johns Hopkins, *Franklin Paine Mall: The Story of a Mind*.

Sabin retired from the Rockefeller Institute in 1938 and moved to Denver, where in 1944 she was named by the governor to a planning committee on postwar public health problems. She drew up a plan and lobbied successfully for a complete reorganization of the state health department. In 1948 she was appointed head of the Denver health department and served in that post until resigning in 1953. She died a short time later that year, and the state of Colorado subsequently chose her as one of its two representatives in Statuary Hall of the U.S. Capitol.

SARA JOSEPHINE BAKER
(born Nov. 15, 1873, Poughkeepsie, N.Y., U.S.–died Feb. 22, 1945, New York, N.Y.)

Sara Josephine Baker was an American physician who contributed significantly to public health and child welfare in the United States.

Baker prepared at private schools for Vassar College, but the death of her father put that school out of reach. She decided to study medicine and after a year of private preparation entered the Women's Medical College of the New York Infirmary in New York City. After graduating in 1898 she interned at the New England Hospital for Women and Children and then entered private practice in New York City.

In 1901 Baker was appointed a medical inspector for the city health department, and in 1907 she became assistant to the commissioner of health. In that post she aided in the apprehension of "Typhoid Mary" Mallon. More importantly, however, she developed from the rudimentary program of inspection for infectious diseases a comprehensive approach to preventive health care for children. In the summer of 1908 she was allowed to test her plan in a slum district on the East Side. A team of 30 nurses under her direction sought out every infant in the district, taught simple hygiene—ventilation, bathing, light clothing, breast-feeding—to the mothers, and made follow-up visits. At the end of the summer the district had recorded 1,200 fewer cases of infant mortality than the previous summer.

In August 1908 the Division of Child Hygiene was established in the health department and Baker was named

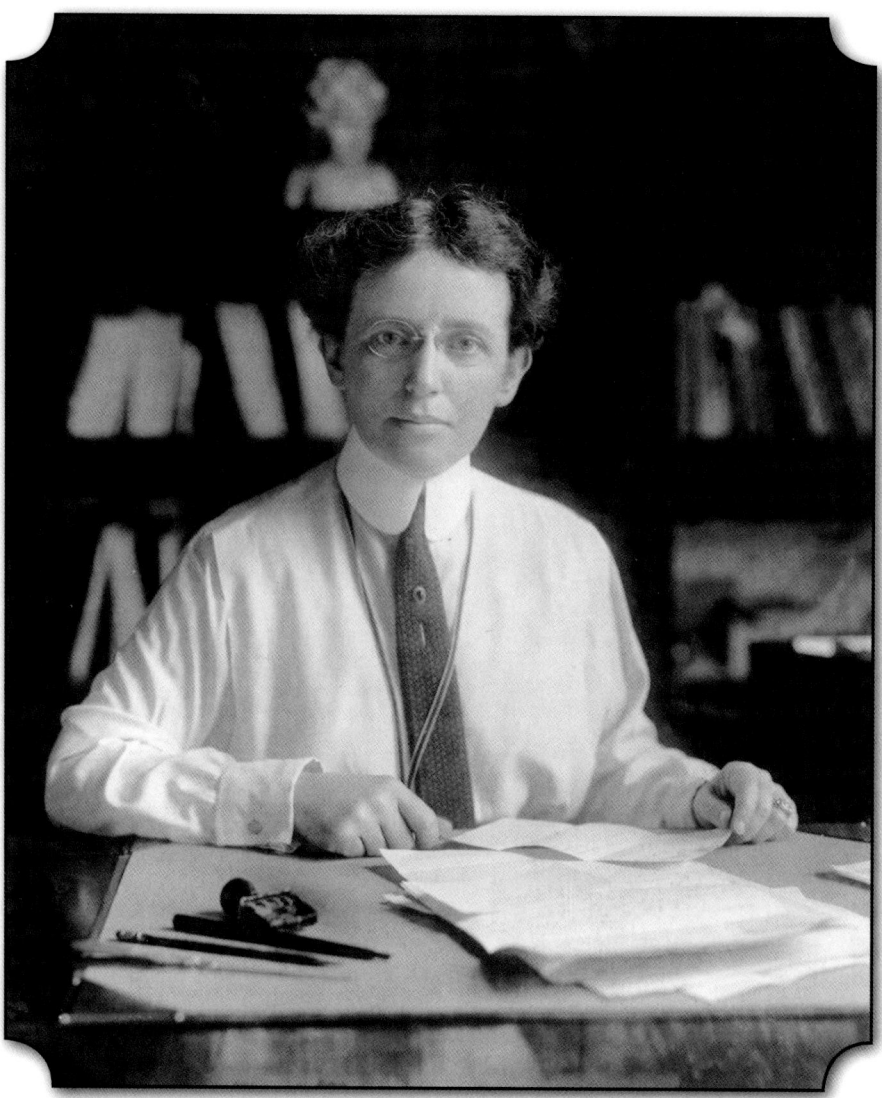

Sara Josephine Baker was a seminal figure in the advancement of child welfare and health in the United States.

director. The division (later raised to bureau) was the first government agency in the world devoted to child health. There Baker evolved a broad program including strict examination and licensing of midwives (and from 1911 free instruction at Bellevue Hospital), appointment of school nurses and doctors, compulsory use of silver nitrate drops in the eyes of all newborns, inspection of schoolchildren for infectious diseases, and numerous methods of distributing information on health and hygiene among the poor.

To deal with the inescapable problem faced by working mothers, Baker organized "Little Mothers' Leagues" to provide training to young girls required to care for infants. In 1911 she organized and became president of the Babies Welfare Association; the next year it was reorganized as the Children's Welfare Federation of New York, of which she was president until 1914 and chairman of the executive committee in 1914–17. As a result of her division's work, the infant mortality rate in New York City fell from 144 per 1,000 live births in 1908 to 88 in 1918 and 66 in 1923. By that time the division's health stations were caring for some 60,000 babies a year—half those born in the city. From 1916 to 1930 she lectured on child hygiene at the New York University-Bellevue Hospital Medical School, and in 1917 she was the first woman to receive from it a doctorate in public health. For 16 years, from its organization in 1912, she was a staff consultant to the federal Children's Bureau. After her retirement from the Bureau of Child Hygiene in 1923, she became a consultant to the Children's Bureau and a representative on child health issues to the League of Nations.

In addition to articles in popular and professional journals, Baker published *Healthy Babies*, *Healthy Children*, and *Healthy Mothers* (all 1920), *The Growing Child* (1923), *Child Hygiene* (1925), and an autobiography, *Fighting for Life* (1939).

CARL JUNG
(born July 26, 1875, Kesswil, Switzerland–died June 6, 1961, Küsnacht)

Carl Jung (in full Carl Gustav Jung) was a Swiss psychologist and psychiatrist who founded analytic psychology, in some aspects a response to Sigmund Freud's psychoanalysis. Jung proposed and developed the concepts of the extraverted and the introverted personality, archetypes, and the collective unconscious. His work has been influential in psychiatry and in the study of religion, literature, and related fields.

Early Life and Career

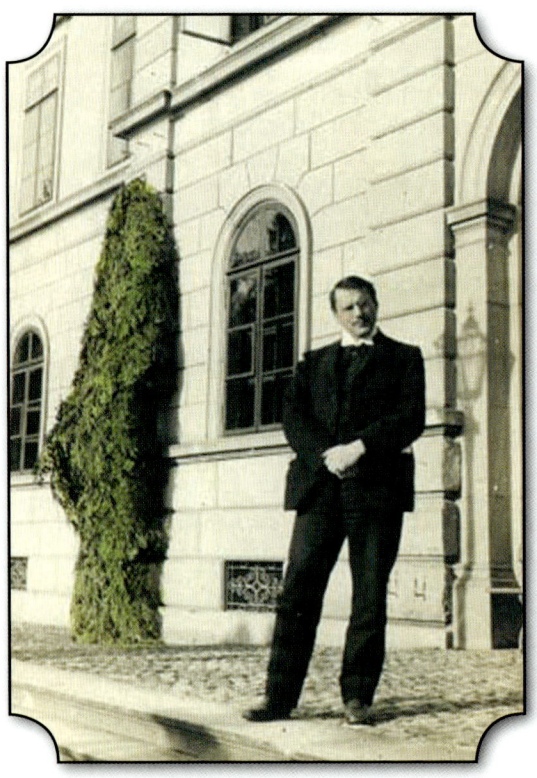

Carl Jung is seen here in front of the Burghölzli Asylum in Zürich, where he served on staff, c. 1909.

Jung was the son of a philologist and pastor. His childhood was lonely, although enriched by a vivid imagination, and from an early age he observed the behaviour of his parents and teachers, which he tried to resolve. Especially concerned with his father's failing belief in religion, he tried to communicate to him his own experience of God. In many ways, the elder Jung was a kind and tolerant man, but neither he nor his son succeeded in understanding each other. Jung seemed destined to become a minister, for there were a number of clergymen on both sides of his family. In his teens he discovered philosophy and read widely, and this, together with the disappointments of his boyhood, led him to forsake the strong family tradition and to study medicine and become a psychiatrist. He was a student at the universities of Basel (1895–1900) and Zürich (M.D., 1902).

He was fortunate in joining the staff of the Burghölzli Asylum of the University of Zürich at a time (1900) when it was under the direction of Eugen Bleuler, whose psychological interests had initiated what are now considered classical studies of mental illness. At Burghölzli, Jung began, with outstanding success, to apply association tests initiated by earlier researchers. He studied, especially, patients' peculiar and illogical responses to stimulus words and found that they were caused by emotionally charged clusters of associations withheld from consciousness because of their disagreeable, immoral (to them), and frequently sexual content. He used the now famous term *complex* to describe such conditions.

Association with Freud

These researches, which established him as a psychiatrist of international repute, led him to understand Freud's investigations; his findings confirmed many of Freud's ideas, and, for a period of five years (between 1907 and 1912), he was Freud's close collaborator. He held important positions in the psychoanalytic movement and was widely thought of as the most likely successor to the founder of psychoanalysis. But this was not to be the outcome of their relationship. Partly for temperamental reasons and partly because of differences of viewpoint, the collaboration ended. At this stage Jung differed with Freud largely over the latter's insistence on the sexual bases of neurosis. A serious disagreement came in 1912, with the publication of Jung's *Wandlungen und Symbole der Libido* (*Psychology of the Unconscious*, 1916), which ran counter to many of Freud's ideas. Although Jung had been elected president of the International Psychoanalytic Society in 1911, he resigned from the society in 1914.

His first achievement was to differentiate two classes of people according to attitude types: extraverted (outward-looking) and introverted (inward-looking). Later he differentiated four functions of the mind—thinking, feeling, sensation, and intuition—one or more of which predominate in any given person. Results of this study were embodied in *Psychologische Typen* (1921; *Psychological Types*, 1923). Jung's wide scholarship was well manifested here, as it also had been in *The Psychology of the Unconscious.*

As a boy Jung had remarkably striking dreams and powerful fantasies that had developed with unusual intensity. After his break with Freud, he deliberately allowed this aspect of himself to function again and gave the irrational side of his nature free expression. At the same time, he studied it scientifically by keeping detailed notes of his strange experiences. He later developed the theory that these experiences came from an area of the mind that he called the collective unconscious, which he held was shared by everyone. This much-contested conception was combined with a theory of archetypes that Jung held as fundamental to the study of the psychology of religion. In Jung's terms, archetypes are instinctive patterns, have a universal character, and are expressed in behaviour and images.

Character of His Psychotherapy

Jung devoted the rest of his life to developing his ideas, especially those on the relation between psychology and religion. In his view, obscure and often neglected texts of writers in the past shed unexpected light not only on Jung's own dreams and fantasies but also on those of his patients; he thought it necessary for the successful practice of their art that psychotherapists become familiar with writings of the old masters.

Besides the development of new psychotherapeutic methods that derived from his own experience and the theories developed from them, Jung gave fresh importance to the so-called Hermetic tradition. He conceived that the Christian religion was part of a historic process necessary for the development of consciousness, and he also thought that the heretical movements, starting with Gnosticism and ending in alchemy, were manifestations of unconscious archetypal elements not adequately expressed in the mainstream forms of Christianity. He was particularly impressed with his finding that alchemical-like symbols could be found frequently in modern dreams and fantasies, and he thought that alchemists had constructed a kind of textbook of the collective unconscious. He expounded on this in 4 out of the 18 volumes that make up his *Collected Works*.

His historical studies aided him in pioneering the psychotherapy of the middle-aged and elderly, especially those who felt their lives had lost meaning. He helped them to appreciate the place of their lives in the sequence of history. Most of these patients had lost their religious belief; Jung found that if they could discover their own myth as expressed in dream and imagination they would become more complete personalities. He called this process individuation.

In later years he becam professor of psychology at the Federal Polytechnical University in Zürich (1933–41) and professor of medical psychology at the University of Basel (1943). His personal experience, his continued psychotherapeutic practice, and his wide knowledge of history placed him in a unique position to comment on current events. As early as 1918 he had begun to think that Germany held a special position in Europe; the Nazi revolution was, therefore, highly significant for him, and he delivered a number of hotly contested views that led to his being wrongly branded as a Nazi sympathizer. Jung lived to the age of 85.

The authoritative English collection of all Jung's published writings is Herbert Read, Michael Fordham, and Gerhard Adler (eds.), *The Collected Works of C.G. Jung*, trans. by R.F.C. Hull, 20 vol., 2nd ed. (1966–79). Jung's *The Psychology of the Unconscious* appears in revised form as *Symbols of Transformation* in the *Collected Works*. His other major individual publications include *Über die Psychologie der Dementia Praecox* (1907; *The Psychology of Dementia Praecox*); *Versuch einer Darstellung der psychoanalytischen Theorie* (1913; *The Theory of Psychoanalysis*); *Collected Papers on Analytical Psychology* (1916); *Two Essays on Analytical Psychology* (1928); *Das Geheimnis der goldenen Blüte* (1929; *The Secret of the Golden Flower*); *Modern Man in Search of a Soul* (1933), a collection of essays covering topics from dream analysis and literature to the psychology of religion; *Psychology and Religion* (1938); *Psychologie und Alchemie* (1944; *Psychology and Alchemy*); and *Aion: Untersuchungen zur Symbolgeschichte* (1951; *Aion: Researches into the Phenomenology of the Self*). Jung's *Erinnerungen, Träume, Gedanken* (1962; *Memories, Dreams, Reflections*) is fascinating semiautobiographical reading, partly written by Jung himself and partly recorded by his secretary.

OSWALD AVERY

(born Oct. 21, 1877, Halifax, Nova Scotia, Canada–died Feb. 20, 1955, Nashville, Tenn., U.S.)

Oswald Aver (in full Oswald Theodore Avery) was a Canadian-born American bacteriologist whose research helped ascertain that deoxyribonucleic acid (DNA) is the substance responsible for heredity, thus laying the foundation for the new science of molecular genetics. His work also contributed to the understanding of the chemistry of immunological processes.

Avery received a medical degree from Columbia University College of Physicians and Surgeons in New York City in 1904. After a few years in clinical practice, he joined the Hoagland Laboratory in Brooklyn and turned his attention to bacteriological research. In 1913 he joined the staff of the Rockefeller Institute Hospital in New York City, where he began studying the bacterium responsible for lobar pneumonia, *Streptococcus pneumoniae*, called the pneumococcus. Avery and colleagues isolated a substance in the blood and urine of infected persons that was produced by this bacterium. They identified the substance as a complex carbohydrate called a polysaccharide, which makes up the capsular envelope of the pneumococcus. Based on the recognition that the polysaccharide composition of capsular envelopes can vary, Avery helped classify pneumococci into different types. Avery also found that the polysaccharide could stimulate an immune response — specifically, the production of antibodies — and was the first to demonstrate that a substance other than a protein could do so. The evidence that the polysaccharide composition of a bacterium influences its virulence (ability to cause disease) and its immunological specificity showed that these characteristics can be analyzed biochemically, thus contributing to the development of immunochemistry.

In 1932 Avery turned his attention to an experiment carried out by a British microbiologist named Frederick Griffith. Griffith worked with two strains of *S. pneumoniae* — one encircled by a polysaccharide capsule that was virulent, and another that lacked a capsule and was nonvirulent. Griffith's results showed that the virulent strain could somehow convert, or transform, the nonvirulent strain into an agent of disease. Furthermore, the transformation was heritable — i.e., able to be passed on to succeeding generations of bacteria. Avery, along with many other scientists, set out to determine the chemical nature of the substance that allowed transformation to occur. In 1944 he and his colleagues Maclyn McCarty and Colin MacLeod reported that the transforming substance—the genetic material of the cell—was DNA.

Avery and his research team obtained mixtures from heat-killed virulent bacteria and inactivated either the proteins, polysaccharides (sugar subunits), lipids, DNA, or RNA (ribonucleic acid, a close chemical relative of DNA) and added each type of preparation individually to avirulent cells. The only molecular class whose inactivation prevented transformation to virulence was DNA. Therefore, it seemed that DNA, because it could transform, must be the hereditary material. This result was met initially with skepticism, as many scientists believed that proteins would prove to be the repository of hereditary information. Eventually, however, the role of DNA was proved, and Avery's contribution to genetics was recognized.

MARGARET SANGER
(born Sept. 14, 1879, Corning, N.Y., U.S.–died Sept. 6, 1966, Tucson, Ariz.)

Margaret Sanger (original name Margaret Louisa Higgins) was the founder of the birth-control movement in the United States and an international leader in the field. She is credited with originating the term *birth control*. Like the social movement she founded, the term has been caught up in a quest for acceptance, generating many synonyms: family planning, planned parenthood, responsible parenthood, voluntary parenthood, contraception, fertility regulation, and fertility control.

Sanger was the sixth of 11 children. She attended Claverack College and then took nurse's training in New

York at the White Plains Hospital and the Manhattan Eye and Ear Clinic. She was married twice, to William Sanger in 1900 and, after a divorce, to J. Noah H. Slee in 1922. After a brief teaching career she practiced obstetrical nursing on the Lower East Side of New York City, where she witnessed the relationships between poverty, uncontrolled fertility, high rates of infant and maternal mortality,

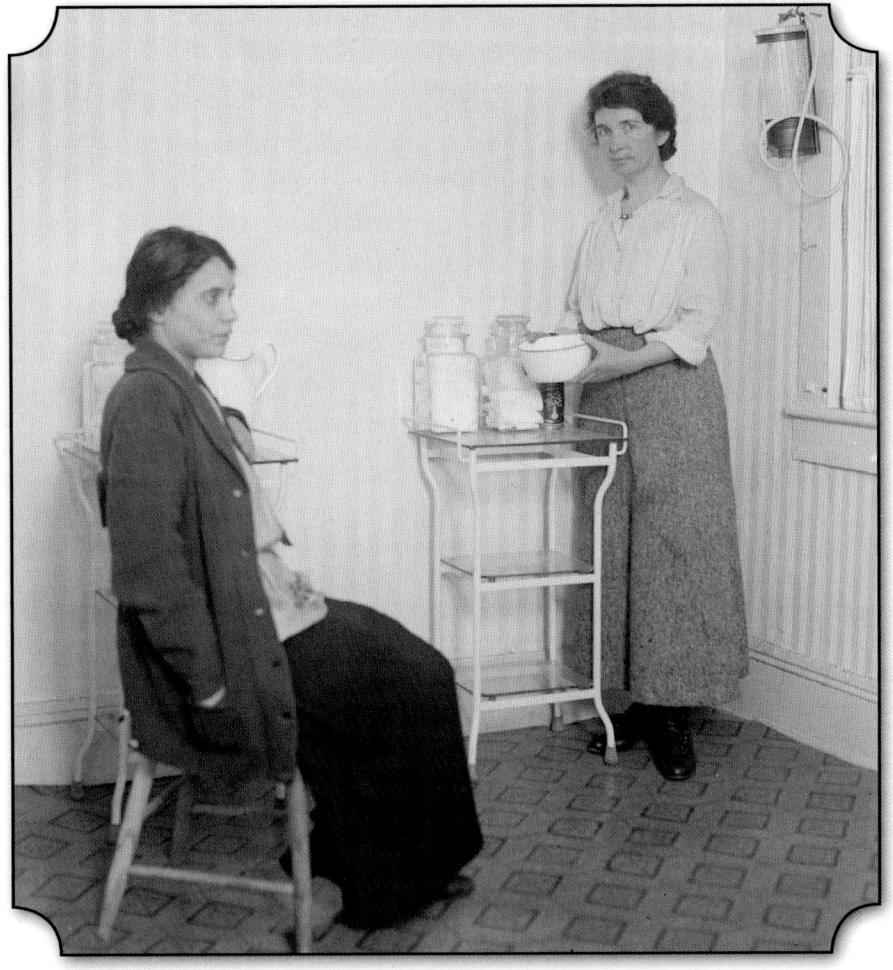

Margaret Sanger is seen here with a client in a family-planning and birth-control clinic.

and deaths from botched illegal abortions. These observations made Sanger a feminist who believed in every woman's right to avoid unwanted pregnancies, and she devoted herself to removing the legal barriers to publicizing the facts about contraception.

In 1912 Sanger gave up nursing to devote herself to the cause of birth control and sex education, publishing a series of articles on the topics, including *What Every Girl Should Know* for the *New York Call*. In 1914 she issued a short-lived magazine, *The Woman Rebel*, and distributed a pamphlet, *Family Limitation*, advocating her views. She was indicted for mailing materials advocating birth control, but the charges were dropped in 1916. Later that year she opened in Brooklyn the first birth-control clinic in the United States. She was arrested and charged with maintaining a "public nuisance," and in 1917 she served 30 days in the Queens penitentiary. While she was serving time, the first issue of her periodical the *Birth Control Review* was published. Her sentencing and subsequent episodes of legal harassment helped to crystallize public opinion in favour of the birth-control movement. Sanger's legal appeals prompted the federal courts first to grant physicians the right to give advice about birth-control methods and then, in 1936, to reinterpret the Comstock Act of 1873 (which had classified contraceptive literature and devices as obscene materials) in such a way as to permit physicians to import and prescribe contraceptives.

In 1921 Sanger founded the American Birth Control League, and she served as its president until 1928. The league was one of the parent organizations of the Birth Control Federation of America, which in 1942 became the Planned Parenthood Federation of America, with Sanger as honorary chairman. Sanger, who had traveled to Europe to study the issue of birth control there, also organized the first World Population Conference in

Geneva in 1927, and she was the first president of the International Planned Parenthood Federation (founded 1953). Subsequently she took her campaign for birth control to Asian countries, especially India and Japan.

Among her numerous books are *What Every Mother Should Know* (1917), *My Fight for Birth Control* (1931), and *Margaret Sanger: An Autobiography* (1938).

MARIE STOPES

(born Oct. 15, 1880, Edinburgh, Scotland–died Oct. 2, 1958, near Dorking, Surrey, England)

Marie Stopes (in full Marie Charlotte Carmichael Stopes) was an advocate of birth control who, in 1921, founded the United Kingdom's first instructional clinic for contraception. Although her clinical work, writings, and speeches evoked violent opposition, especially from Roman Catholics, she greatly influenced the Church of England's gradual relaxation (from 1930) of its stand against birth control.

Stopes grew up in a wealthy, educated family; her father was an architect, her mother a scholar of Shakespeare and an advocate for the education of women. Stopes obtained a science degree (1902) from University College, London, which she completed in only two years. She went on to do postgraduate studies in paleobotany (fossil plants), earning a doctorate from the University of Munich in 1904. That same year she became an assistant lecturer of botany at the University of Manchester. She specialized in fossil plants and the problems of coal mining. She married her first husband, a botanist named Reginald Ruggles Gates, in 1911. Stopes would later assert that her marriage was unconsummated and that she knew little about sex when she first married. Her failed marriage and its eventual annulment in 1916 played a large role in determining her future career, causing her to turn her attention to the issues of sex, marriage, and childbirth and their meaning in society. She initially saw birth control as an aid to marriage fulfillment and as a means to save women from the physical strain of excessive childbearing. In this regard for quality of life of the individual woman, she differed from most other early leaders of the birth-control movement, who were more concerned with social good, such as the elimination of overpopulation and poverty.

In 1918 Stopes married Humphrey Verdon Roe, cofounder of the A.V. Roe aircraft firm, who also had strong interests in the birth-control movement. He helped her in the crusade that she then began. Their original birth-control clinic—designed to educate women about the few methods of birth control available to them—was founded three years later, in the working-class Holloway district of London. That same year she became founder and president of the Society for Constructive Birth Control, a platform from which she spoke widely about the benefits of married women having healthy, desired babies. In the meantime she wrote *Married Love* and *Wise Parenthood* (both 1918), which were widely translated. *Married Love*, an appeal for sexual equality and fulfillment within marriage, was considered to be a radical text at the time. Margaret Sanger met Marie Stopes and persuaded her to add a chapter on birth control. Her *Contraception: Its Theory, History and Practice* (1923) was, when it first appeared, the most comprehensive treatment of the subject. After World War II she promoted birth control in East Asian countries.

ALEXANDER FLEMING

(born Aug. 6, 1881, Lochfield Farm, Darvel, Ayrshire, Scotland–died March 11, 1955, London, England)

Alexander Fleming was a Scottish bacteriologist best known for his discovery of penicillin. Fleming had a genius for technical ingenuity and original observation. His work on wound infection and lysozyme, an antibacterial enzyme found in tears and saliva, guaranteed him a place in the history of bacteriology. But it was his discovery of penicillin in 1928, which started the antibiotic revolution, that sealed his lasting reputation. Fleming was recognized for that achievement in 1945, when he received the Nobel Prize for Physiology or Medicine, along with Australian pathologist Howard Walter Florey and German-born British biochemist Ernst Boris Chain, both of whom isolated and purified penicillin.

Education and Early Career

Fleming was the seventh of eight children of a Scottish hill farmer (third of four children from the farmer's second wife). His country upbringing in southwestern Scotland sharpened his capacities for observation and appreciation of the natural world at an early age. He began his elementary schooling at Loudoun Moor and then moved on to a larger school at Darvel before enrolling in Kilmarnock Academy in 1894. In 1895 he moved to London to live with his elder brother Thomas (who worked as an oculist) and completed his basic education at Regent Street Polytechnic.

After working as a London shipping clerk, Fleming began his medical studies at St. Mary's Hospital Medical School in 1901, funded by a scholarship and a legacy from his uncle. There he won the 1908 gold medal as top medical student at the University of London. At first he planned to become a surgeon, but a temporary position in the laboratories of the Inoculation Department at St. Mary's Hospital convinced him that his future lay in the new field of bacteriology. There he came under the influence of bacteriologist and immunologist Sir Almroth Edward Wright, whose ideas of vaccine therapy seemed to offer a revolutionary direction in medical treatment.

Between 1909 and 1914 Fleming established a successful private practice as a venereologist, and in 1915 he married Sarah Marion McElroy, an Irish nurse. Fleming's son, Robert, born in 1924, followed his father into medicine. Fleming was one of the first doctors in Britain to administer arsphenamine (Salvarsan), a drug effective against syphilis that was discovered by German scientist Paul Ehrlich in 1910. During World War I, Fleming had a commission in the Royal Army Medical Corps and worked as a bacteriologist studying wound infections in a laboratory that Wright had set up in a military hospital housed in a casino in Boulogne, France. There he demonstrated that the use of strong antiseptics on wounds did more harm than good and recommended that the wounds simply be kept clean with a mild saline solution. Fleming returned to St. Mary's after the war and was promoted to assistant director of the Inoculation Department. Years later, in 1946, he succeeded Wright as principal of the department, which was renamed the Wright-Fleming Institute.

In November 1921 Fleming discovered lysozyme, an enzyme present in body fluids such as saliva and tears that has a mild antiseptic effect. That was the first of his major discoveries. It came about when he had a cold and a drop of his nasal mucus fell onto a culture plate of bacteria. Realizing that his mucus might have an effect on bacterial growth, he mixed the mucus into the culture and a few weeks later saw signs of the bacteria's having been dissolved. Fleming's study of lysozyme, which he considered his best work as a scientist, was a significant contribution to the understanding of how the body fights infection. Unfortunately, lysozyme had no effect on the most-pathogenic bacteria.

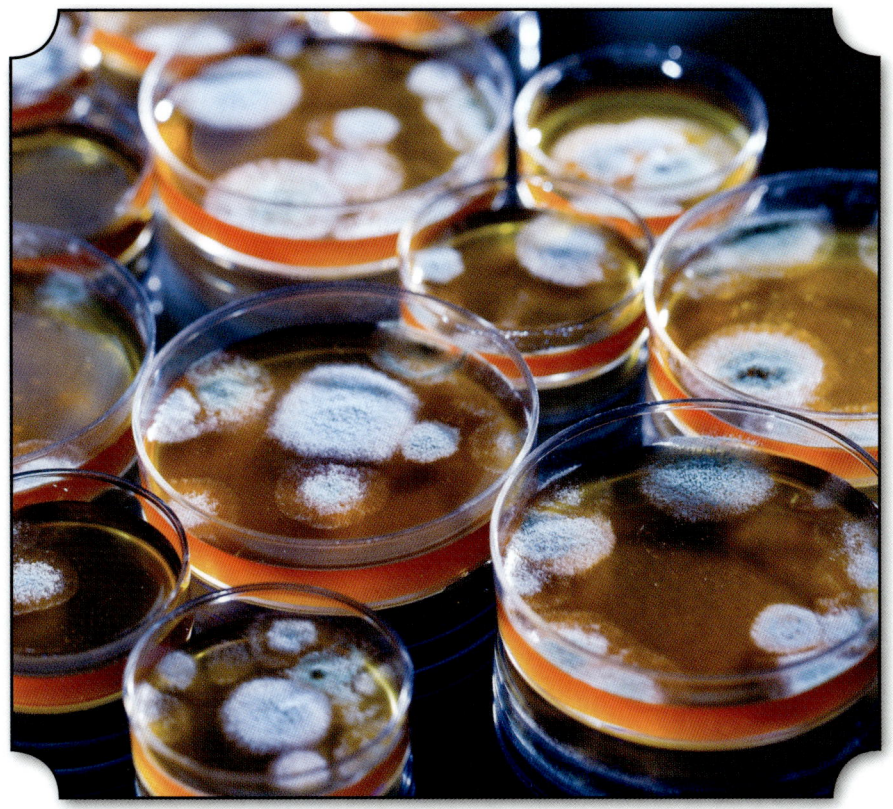

Alexander Fleming's observation of Penicillium notatum *mold, such as that seen here, growing on a culture plate, led to his discovery of penicillin.*

DISCOVERY OF PENICILLIN

On Sept. 3, 1928, shortly after his appointment as professor of bacteriology, Fleming noticed that a culture plate of *Staphylococcus aureus* he had been working on had become contaminated by a fungus. A mold, later identified as *Penicillium notatum* (now classified as *P. chrysogenum*), had inhibited the growth of the bacteria. He at first called the substance "mould juice" and then "penicillin," after the mold that produced it. Fleming decided to investigate further, because he thought that he had found an enzyme more potent than lysozyme. In fact, it was not an enzyme but an antibiotic—one of the first to be discovered. By the time Fleming had established that, he was interested in penicillin for itself. Very much the lone researcher with an eye for the unusual, Fleming had the freedom to pursue anything that interested him. Although that approach was ideal for taking advantage of a chance observation, the therapeutic development of penicillin required multidisciplinary teamwork. Fleming, working with two young researchers, failed to stabilize and purify penicillin. However, he did point out that penicillin had clinical potential, both as a topical antiseptic and as an injectable antibiotic, if it could be isolated and purified.

Penicillin eventually came into use during World War II as the result of the work of a team of scientists led by Howard Florey at the University of Oxford. Though Florey, his coworker Ernst Chain, and Fleming shared the 1945 Nobel Prize, their relationship was clouded owing to the issue of who should gain the most credit for penicillin. Fleming's role was emphasized by the press because of the romance of his chance discovery and his greater willingness to speak to journalists.

Fleming was knighted in 1944. In 1949 his first wife, who had changed her name to Sareen, died. In 1953, two years prior to his death, Fleming married Greek microbiologist Amalia Coutsouris-Voureka, who had been involved in the Greek resistance movement during World War II and had been Fleming's colleague since 1946, when she enrolled at St. Mary's Hospital on a scholarship. For the last decade of his life, Fleming was feted universally for his discovery of penicillin and acted as a world ambassador for medicine and science. Initially a shy uncommunicative man and a poor lecturer, he blossomed under the attention he received, becoming one of the world's best-known scientists.

SELMAN ABRAHAM WAKSMAN
(born July 22, 1888, Priluka, Ukraine, Russian Empire [now Pryluky, Ukraine]–died Aug. 16, 1973, Hyannis, Mass., U.S.)

Selman Abraham Waksman was a Ukrainian-born American biochemist who was one of the world's foremost authorities on soil microbiology. After the discovery of penicillin, he played a major role in initiating a calculated, systematic search for antibiotics among microbes. His screening methods and consequent codiscovery of the antibiotic streptomycin, the first specific agent effective in the treatment of tuberculosis, brought him the 1952 Nobel Prize for Physiology or Medicine.

A naturalized U.S. citizen (1916), Waksman spent most of his career at Rutgers University, New Brunswick, N.J., where he served as professor of soil microbiology (1930–40), professor of microbiology and chairman of the department (1940–58), and director of the Rutgers Institute of Microbiology (1949–58). During his extensive study of the actinomycetes (filamentous, bacteria-like microorganisms found in the soil), he extracted from them antibiotics (a term he coined in 1941) valuable for their killing effect not only on gram-positive bacteria, such as the tubercle bacillus (*Mycobacterium tuberculosis*, which unlike other gram-positive microbes is insensitive to penicillin), but also on gram-negative bacteria, such as the organisms that cause cholera (*Vibrio cholerae*) and typhoid fever (*Salmonella typhi*).

In 1940 Waksman, along with his graduate student H. Boyd Woodruff, isolated actinomycin from soil bacteria.

Although the substance was effective against strains of gram-negative and gram-positive bacteria, including *M. tuberculosis*, it was extremely toxic when given to test animals. Four years later Waksman and graduate students Albert Schatz and Elizabeth Bugie published a paper describing their discovery of the relatively nontoxic streptomycin, which they extracted from the actinomycete *Streptomyces griseus*. They found that the antibiotic exercised repressive influence on tuberculosis. In combination with other chemotherapeutic agents, streptomycin has become a major factor in controlling the disease. Waksman also isolated and developed several other antibiotics, including neomycin, that have been used in treating many infectious diseases of humans, domestic animals, and plants.

Among Waksman's books are *Principles of Soil Microbiology* (1927), regarded as one of the most exhaustive works on the subject, and *My Life with the Microbes* (1954), an autobiography.

FREDERICK GRANT BANTING
(born Nov. 14, 1891, Alliston, Ontario, Canada–died Feb. 21, 1941, Newfoundland)

Sir Frederick Grant Banting was a Canadian physician who, with Charles H. Best, was one of the first to extract (1921) the hormone insulin from the pancreas. Injections of insulin proved to be the first effective treatment for diabetes, a disease in which glucose accumulates in abnormally high quantities in the blood. Banting was awarded a share of the 1923 Nobel Prize for Physiology or Medicine for his achievement.

Banting was educated at the University of Toronto, served in World War I, and then practiced medicine in London, Ontario. In 1889 Joseph von Mering and Oskar

Minkowski had found that complete removal of the pancreas in dogs immediately caused severe diabetes. Later scientists hypothesized that the pancreas controlled glucose metabolism by generating a hormone, which they named "insulin." However, repeated efforts to extract insulin from the pancreas ended in failure, because the pancreas' own digestive enzymes destroyed the insulin molecules as soon as the pancreas was ground up.

In May 1921 Banting and Best, a medical student, began an intensive effort in the laboratories of the Scottish physiologist J.J.R. Macleod, at the University of Toronto, to isolate the hormone. By tying off the pancreatic ducts of dogs, they were able to reduce the pancreas to inactivity while preserving certain cells in the pancreas known as the islets of Langerhans, which were thought to be the site of insulin production. Solutions extracted from these cells were injected into the dogs whose pancreas had been removed, and the dogs quickly recovered from their artificially induced diabetes. Banting and Best were able to isolate insulin in a form that proved consistently effective in treating diabetes in humans. This discovery ultimately enabled millions of people suffering from diabetes to lead normal lives.

Banting and Best completed their experiments in 1922. The following year Banting and Macleod received the 1923 Nobel Prize for Physiology or Medicine for the discovery of insulin, though Macleod had not actually taken part in the original research. Angered that Macleod, rather than Best, had received the Nobel Prize, Banting divided his share of the award equally with Best. Macleod shared his portion of the Nobel Prize with James B. Collip, a young chemist who had helped with the purification of insulin. In 1923 Banting became head of the University of Toronto's Banting and Best Department of Medical Research. Banting was created a knight of the British Empire in 1934. He was killed in a plane crash in 1941 while on a war mission.

HELEN BROOKE TAUSSIG
(born May 24, 1898, Cambridge, Mass., U.S.–died May 20, 1986, Kennett Square, Pa.)

Helen Brooke Taussig was an American physician recognized as the founder of pediatric cardiology, best known for her contributions to the development of the first successful treatment of "blue baby" syndrome.

Helen Taussig was born into a distinguished family as the daughter of Frank and Edith Guild Taussig. Her father was a prominent economics professor at Harvard University, and her mother was one of the first women to attend Radcliffe College (today known as the Radcliffe Institute for Advanced Study), an extension of Harvard that provided instruction for women. Although Taussig enjoyed a privileged upbringing, adversity cultivated in her a determination that later defined her character. As a child, the dyslexic Taussig laboured to become proficient in reading and was tutored by her father, who recognized the potential of her logical mind. When Taussig was 11, her mother died of tuberculosis, an illness Helen would later contract as well. However, these obstacles did not discourage Taussig from obtaining a university education. She enrolled at Radcliffe College in 1917, transferring to the University of California, Berkeley, in 1919, where she earned an A.B. in 1921. Taussig aspired to study medicine at Harvard but was denied admission because the university did not accept women into its academic degree program. Instead, she attended the Boston University School of Medicine from 1922 to 1924 and graduated from the Johns Hopkins University School of Medicine in 1927.

Two individuals had a far-reaching impact on Taussig's career. First was Canadian pathologist Maude Abbott of McGill University in Montreal. Abbott was a strong-minded role model whose earlier studies of congenital heart disease created the foundation for Taussig's own research into heart disease. Then, while an intern at Johns Hopkins, Taussig's work attracted the attention of American pediatrician Edwards A. Park, the director and, later, the chief of pediatrics at Johns Hopkins. In 1930 Park elevated Taussig to director of Hopkins' Harriet Lane Clinic, a health care centre for children, making her one of the first women in the country to hold such a prestigious position.

Taussig's career advanced, but her personal challenges mounted. In her 30s she grew deaf, and as a result she developed an innovative method to explore the beat of the human heart using her hands to compensate for her hearing loss. Relying on this method, Taussig noticed common beat patterns in the malformed hearts of infant patients who outwardly displayed a cyanotic hue and hence were known as "blue babies." She traced the root of the problem to a lack of oxygenated blood circulating from the lungs to the heart. Taussig reasoned that the creation of an arterial patent ductus, or shunt, would alleviate the problem, and she championed the cause before American surgeon Alfred Blalock, Hopkins' chief of the department of surgery. Together they developed the Blalock-Taussig shunt, an artery-like tube designed to deliver oxygen-rich blood from the lungs to the heart. On Nov. 29, 1944, Eileen Saxton, an infant affected by tetralogy of Fallot, a congenital heart disorder that gives rise to blue baby syndrome and that was previously considered untreatable, became the first patient to survive a successfully implanted Blalock-Taussig shunt. The miracle surgery was touted in the American magazines *Time* and *Life*, as well as in newspapers around the world. Later, American laboratory technician Vivien Thomas was also recognized for his contributions to the surgery.

Taussig was a prolific writer, publishing an astounding number of medical papers. In 1947 she wrote *Congenital Malformations of the Heart*, which was revised in 1960. Throughout her lifetime she received worldwide honours. She was awarded the Medal of Freedom by U.S. Pres. Lyndon B. Johnson in 1964, and in 1965 Taussig became the first woman president of the American Heart Association. In addition, Taussig testified before the U.S. Congress about the harmful effects of the drug thalidomide, which had produced deformed children in Europe.

Taussig's ideas and determination have had long-lasting impacts on cardiology. Physicians originally believed the early blue babies could possibly endure a 40-year life span. At the turn of the 21st century, some of these early patients continued to survive into their sixth decade.

HOWARD WALTER FLOREY

(born Sept. 24, 1898, Adelaide, Australia–died Feb. 21, 1968, Oxford, England)

Howard Walter Florey, Baron Florey, was an Australian pathologist who, with Ernst Boris Chain, isolated and purified penicillin (discovered in 1928 by Sir Alexander Fleming) for general clinical use. For this research Florey,

Chain, and Fleming shared the Nobel Prize for Physiology or Medicine in 1945.

Florey studied medicine at Adelaide and Oxford universities until 1924. After holding teaching and research posts at Cambridge and Sheffield universities, he was professor of pathology at Oxford (1935–62). He was appointed provost of Queen's College, Oxford (1962), and chancellor of the Australian National University, Canberra (1965), positions he held until his death. He also served as president of the Royal Society (1960–65). He was knighted in 1944 and made life peer, assuming his title as baron, in 1965. Florey investigated tissue inflammation and secretion of mucous membranes. He succeeded in purifying lysozyme, a bacteria-destroying enzyme found in tears and saliva, and characterized the substances acted upon by the enzyme. In 1939 he surveyed other naturally occurring antibacterial substances, concentrating on penicillin. With Chain and others, he demonstrated its curative properties in human studies and developed methods for its production. Following World War II and the work of his research team in North Africa, penicillin came into widespread clinical use.

CHARLES BEST

(born Feb. 27, 1899, West Pembroke, Maine, U.S.–died March 31, 1978, Toronto, Ontario, Canada)

Charles Best (in full Charles Herbert Best) was a physiologist who, with Sir Frederick Banting, was one of the first to obtain (1921) a pancreatic extract of insulin in a form that controlled diabetes in dogs. The successful use of insulin in treating human patients followed. But because Best did not receive his medical degree until 1925, he did not share the Nobel Prize for Physiology or Medicine awarded to Banting and J.J.R. Macleod in 1923 for their role in the work. Best also discovered the vitamin choline and the enzyme histaminase. He was one of the first to introduce anticoagulants in treatment of thrombosis (blood clots).

In May 1921, while still an undergraduate, Best became a laboratory assistant to Banting at the University of Toronto. In the months that followed, they performed their prizewinning research on insulin. Best continued as research associate in the Banting and Best Department of Medical Research, which was created at the university in 1923, and he succeeded Banting as its director (1941–67). With Banting he wrote *Internal Secretions of the Pancreas* (1922).

ALFRED BLALOCK

(born April 5, 1899, Culloden, Ga., U.S.–died Sept. 15, 1964, Baltimore, Md.)

Alfred Blalock was an American surgeon who, with pediatric cardiologist Helen B. Taussig, devised a surgical treatment for infants born with the condition known as the tetralogy of Fallot, or "blue baby" syndrome.

After graduating from the University of Georgia in 1918 Blalock entered the Johns Hopkins University School of Medicine, from which he received his M.D. degree in 1922. From 1925 to 1941 he was a resident in surgery in the school of medicine of Vanderbilt University. During that time he conducted research on traumatic and hemorrhagic shock; his conclusion that the effects of shock were due to loss of blood volume led to the volume-replacement treatment that was credited with saving countless lives during World War II.

Blalock returned to Johns Hopkins in 1941 as professor and head of the department of surgery in the school of medicine and as surgeon-in-chief of the Johns Hopkins Hospital. In collaboration with Taussig, Blalock devised a procedure known as subclavian-pulmonary artery anastomosis, by which the congenital heart defect that produced the "blue baby" syndrome could be corrected and the patient enabled to lead a nearly normal life. The first such operation was performed by Blalock in 1944.

PERCY JULIAN

(born April 11, 1899, Montgomery, Ala., U.S.–died April 19, 1975, Waukegan, Ill.)

Percy Julian (in full Percy Lavon Julian) was an American chemist, synthesist of cortisone, hormones, and other products from soybeans.

Percy Julian attended De Pauw University (A.B., 1920) and Harvard University (M.A., 1923) and studied under Ernst Späth, who synthesized nicotine and ephedrine, at the University of Vienna (Ph.D., 1931). Julian also taught chemistry at Fisk University, West Virginia State College for Negroes, and Howard and De Pauw universities before, in 1936, directing research into soybeans at the Glidden Company in Chicago. He became director of chemicals development there before leaving in 1953 to found his own companies.

In his researches Julian isolated simple compounds in natural products, then investigated how those compounds were naturally altered into chemicals essential to life, including vitamins and hormones; he then attempted to create the compounds artificially. Early in his career Julian attracted attention for synthesizing the drug physostigmine, used to treat glaucoma. He refined a soya protein that became the basis of Aero-Foam, a foam fire extinguisher used by the U.S. Navy in World War II. He led research that resulted in quantity production of the hormones progesterone (female) and testosterone (male) and of cortisone drugs.

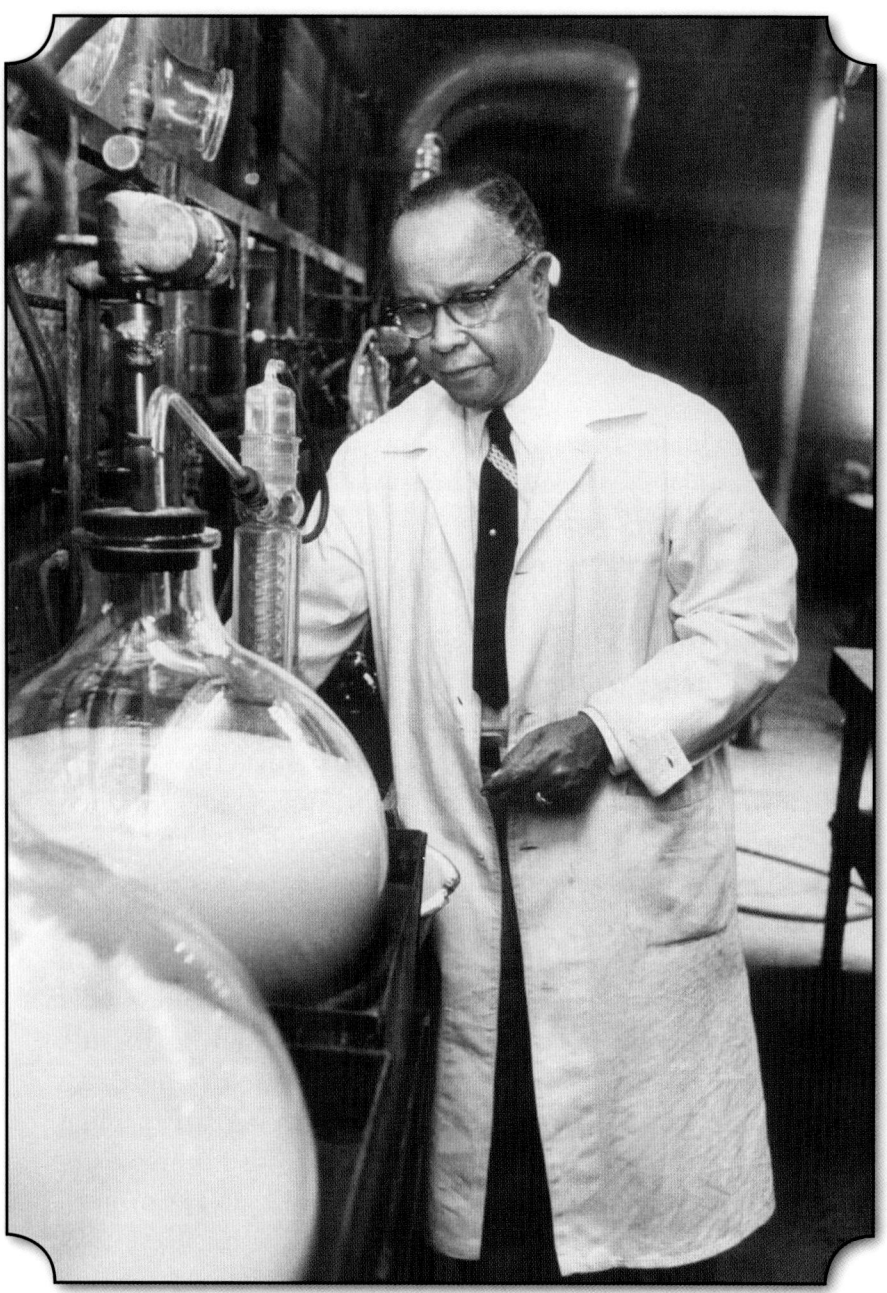

Although he was a chemist by training, Percy Julian's work was instrumental in the development of various medical breakthroughs.

In 1950 Julian, an African American, was named Chicago's Man of the Year in a *Chicago Sun-Times* poll, but his home was bombed and burned when he moved to the all-white suburb of Oak Park. He was active as a fundraiser for the National Association for the Advancement of Colored People (NAACP) for their project to sue to enforce civil rights legislation.

BARBARA MCCLINTOCK
(born June 16, 1902, Hartford, Conn., U.S.–died Sept. 2, 1992, Huntington, N.Y.)

Barbara McClintock was an American scientist whose discovery in the 1940s and '50s of mobile genetic elements, or "jumping genes," won her the Nobel Prize for Physiology or Medicine in 1983.

McClintock, whose father was a physician, took great pleasure in science as a child and evidenced early the independence of mind and action that she would exhibit throughout the rest of her life. After attending high school, she enrolled as a biology major at Cornell University in 1919. She received a B.S. in 1923, a master's degree two years later, and, having specialized in cytology, genetics, and zoology, a Ph.D. in 1927. During graduate school she began the work that would occupy her entire professional life: the chromosomal analysis of corn (maize). She used a microscope and a staining technique that allowed her to examine, identify, and describe individual corn chromosomes.

In 1931 she and a colleague, Harriet Creighton, published "A Correlation of Cytological and Genetical Crossing-over in *Zea mays*," a paper that established that chromosomes formed the basis of genetics. Based on her experiments and publications during the 1930s, McClintock was elected vice president of the Genetics

Society of America in 1939 and president of the Genetics Society in 1944. She received a Guggenheim Fellowship in 1933 to study in Germany, but she left early because of the rise of Nazism. When she returned to Cornell, her alma mater, she found that the university would not hire a female professor. The Rockefeller Foundation funded her research at Cornell (1934–36) until she was hired by the University of Missouri (1936–41).

In 1941 McClintock moved to Long Island, N.Y., to work at the Cold Spring Harbor Laboratory, where she spent the rest of her professional life. In the 1940s, by observing and experimenting with variations in the coloration of kernels of corn, she discovered that genetic information is not stationary. By tracing pigmentation changes in corn and using a microscope to examine that plant's large chromosomes, she isolated two genes that she called "controlling elements." These genes controlled the genes that were actually responsible for pigmentation. McClintock found that the controlling elements could move along the chromosome to a different site, and that these changes affected the behaviour of neighbouring genes. She suggested that these transposable elements were responsible for new mutations in pigmentation or other characteristics. Although these elements are frequently called "jumping genes," they are always maintained in an integrated site in the genome. In addition, most of the "jumping genes" (transposons) eventually become inactive and no longer move.

McClintock's work was ahead of its time and was for many years considered too radical—or was simply ignored—by her fellow scientists. Deeply disappointed with her colleagues, she stopped publishing the results of her work and ceased giving lectures, though she continued doing research. Not until the late 1960s and '70s, after biologists had determined that the genetic material was DNA, did members of the scientific community begin to verify her early findings. When recognition finally came, McClintock was inundated with awards and honours, most notably the 1983 Nobel Prize for Physiology or Medicine. She was the first woman to be the sole winner of this award.

CHARLES RICHARD DREW

(born June 3, 1904, Washington, D.C., U.S.–died April 1, 1950, near Burlington, N.C.)

Charles Richard Drew was an African American physician and surgeon who was an authority on the preservation of human blood for transfusion.

Drew was educated at Amherst College (graduated 1926), McGill University, Montreal (1933), and Columbia University (1940). While earning his doctorate at Columbia in the late 1930s, he conducted research into the properties and preservation of blood plasma. He soon developed efficient ways to process and store large quantities of blood plasma in "blood banks." As the leading authority in the field, he organized and directed the blood-plasma programs of the United States and Great Britain in the early years of World War II, while also agitating the authorities to stop excluding the blood of African Americans from plasma-supply networks.

Drew resigned his official posts in 1942 after the armed forces ruled that the blood of African Americans would be accepted but would have to be stored separately from that of whites. He then became a surgeon and professor of medicine at Freedmen's Hospital, Washington, D.C., and Howard University (1942–50).

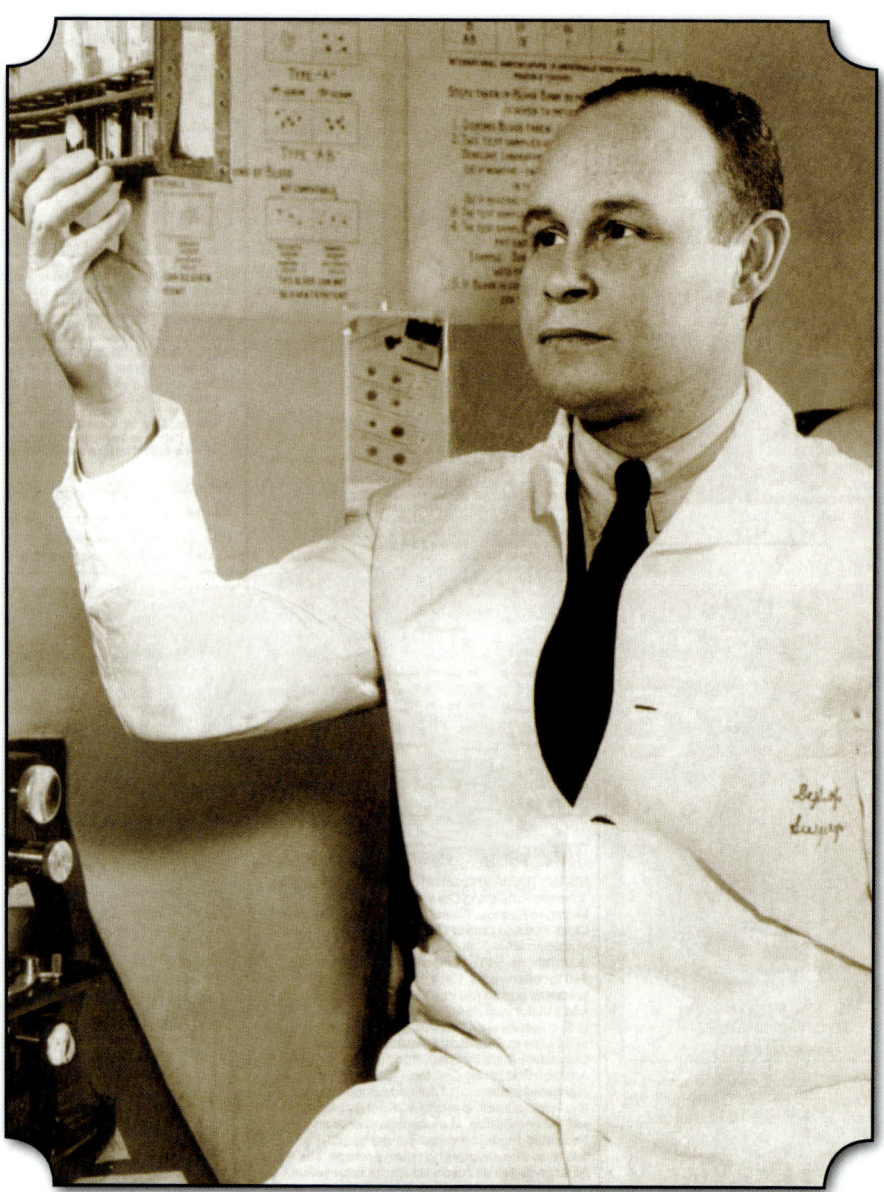

In addition to his work in blood preservation and transfusion, Charles Drew served as the first black surgeon examiner of the American Board of Surgery.

He was fatally injured in an automobile accident in 1950.

ERNST BORIS CHAIN
(born June 19, 1906, Berlin, Germany–died Aug. 12, 1979, Mulrany, Ireland)

Sir Ernst Boris Chain was a German-born British biochemist who, with pathologist Howard Walter Florey (later Baron Florey), isolated and purified penicillin (which had been discovered in 1928 by Sir Alexander Fleming) and performed the first clinical trials of the antibiotic. For their pioneering work on penicillin Chain, Florey, and Fleming shared the 1945 Nobel Prize for Physiology or Medicine.

Chain graduated in chemistry and physiology from the Friedrich Wilhelm University of Berlin and then engaged in research at the Institute of Pathology, Charité Hospital, Berlin (1930–33). Forced to flee Germany because of the anti-Semitic policies of Adolf Hitler, he went first to the University of Cambridge, working under Sir Frederick G. Hopkins, and then (1935) to the University of Oxford, where he worked with Florey on penicillin.

Chain served as the director of the International Research Centre for Chemical Microbiology, Superior Institute of Health, Rome, from 1948 until 1961. He then joined the faculty of Imperial College, University of London, where he was professor of biochemistry (1961–73), professor emeritus and senior research fellow (1973–76), and fellow (1978–79). Chain was knighted in 1969.

In addition to his work on antibiotics, Chain studied snake venoms; the spreading factor, an enzyme that facilitates the dispersal of fluids in tissue; and insulin.

ALBERT SABIN

(born Aug. 26, 1906, Bialystok, Poland, Russian Empire–died March 3, 1993, Washington, D.C., U.S.)

Albert Sabin was a Polish American physician and microbiologist best known for developing the oral polio vaccine. He was also known for his research in the fields of human viral diseases, toxoplasmosis, and cancer.

Sabin immigrated with his parents to the United States in 1921 and became an American citizen nine years later. He received an M.D. degree from New York University in 1931, where he began research on human poliomyelitis. After serving for two years as a house physician at Bellevue Hospital in New York City, he attended the Lister Institute of Preventive Medicine in London. In 1935 he joined the staff of the Rockefeller Institute for Medical Research in New York City, where he was the first researcher to demonstrate the growth of poliovirus in human nervous tissue outside the body.

In 1939 Sabin became associate professor of pediatrics at the University of Cincinnati College of Medicine in Ohio and chief of the division of infectious diseases at the Children's Hospital Research Foundation of the college. He later became professor of research pediatrics. While at the college, he disproved the prevailing theory that the poliovirus enters the body through the nose and respiratory system; he subsequently demonstrated that human poliomyelitis is primarily an infection of the digestive tract.

The first polio vaccine, known as inactivated poliovirus vaccine (IPV) or Salk vaccine, was developed in the early 1950s by American physician Jonas Salk. This vaccine contains killed virus and is given by injection. Sabin postulated that live, weakened (attenuated) virus, administered orally, would provide immunity over a longer period of time than killed, injected virus. By 1957 he had isolated strains of each of the three types of poliovirus that were not strong enough to produce the disease itself but were capable of stimulating the production of antibodies. He then proceeded to conduct preliminary experiments in the oral administration of these attenuated strains. Cooperative studies were conducted with scientists from Mexico, the Netherlands, and the Soviet Union, and finally, in extensive field trials on children, the effectiveness of the new vaccine was conclusively demonstrated. The Sabin oral polio vaccine was approved for use in the United States in 1960 and became the main defense against polio throughout the world.

Sabin also isolated the B virus, conducted research that led to the development of vaccines for sandfly fever and dengue, studied how immunity to viruses is developed, investigated viruses that affect the nervous system, and studied the role of viruses in cancer.

Sabin became professor emeritus at Cincinnati in 1971, and from 1974 to 1982 he was a research professor at the Medical University of South Carolina in Charleston.

RITA LEVI-MONTALCINI

(born April 22, 1909, Turin, Italy–died Dec. 30, 2012, Rome)

Rita Levi-Montalcini was an Italian American neurologist who, with biochemist Stanley Cohen, shared the Nobel Prize for Physiology or Medicine in 1986 for her discovery of a bodily substance that stimulates and influences the growth of nerve cells.

Levi-Montalcini studied medicine at the University of Turin and did research there on the effects that peripheral tissues have on nerve cell growth. Although she was forced into hiding in Florence during the German occupation of Italy (1943–45) because of her Jewish ancestry, she was able to resume her research at Turin after the war. In 1947 she

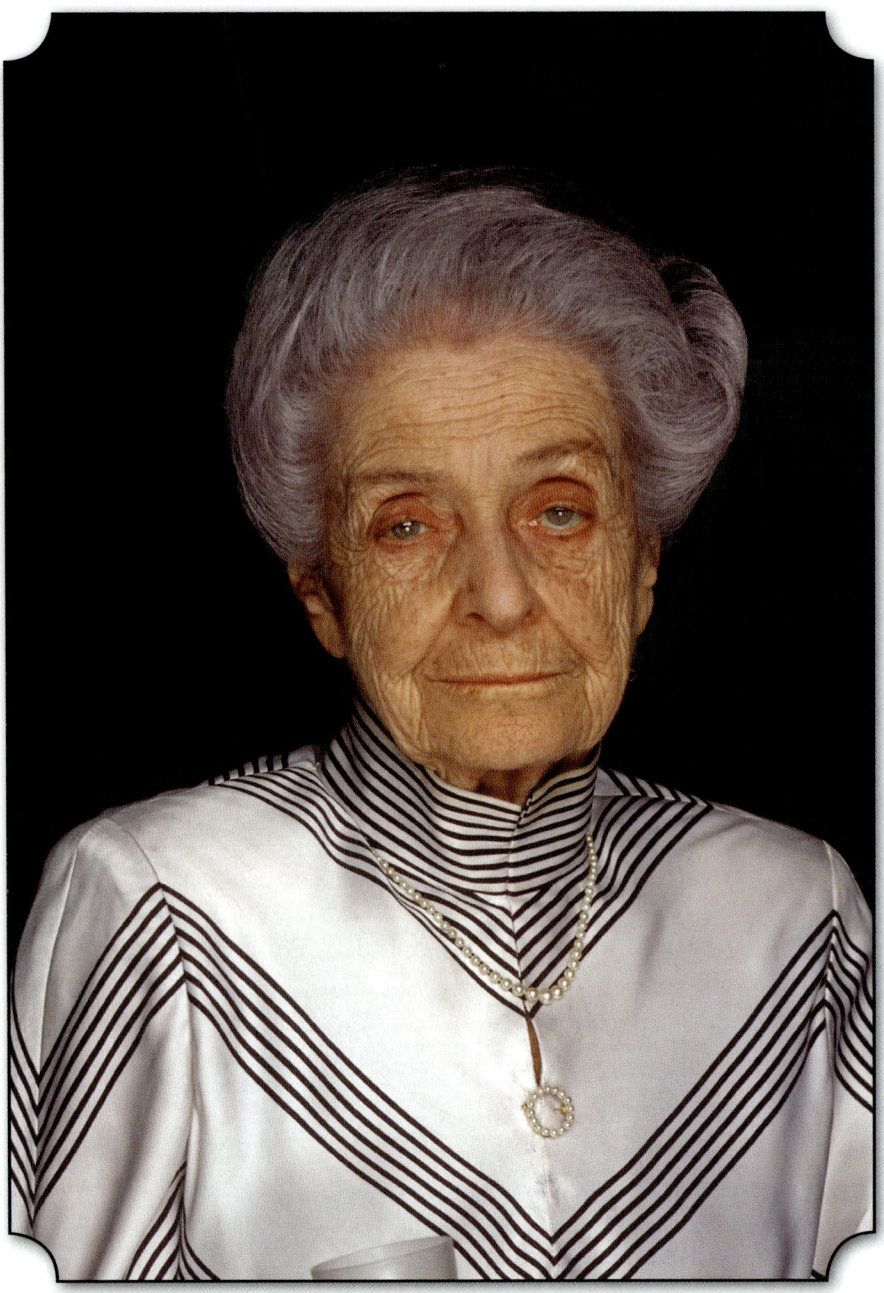

The work of Rita Levi-Montalcini helped advance scientific understanding of diseases such as cancer and Alzheimer disease.

accepted a post at Washington University, St. Louis, Mo., with the zoologist Viktor Hamburger, who was studying the growth of nerve tissue in chick embryos. She eventually held dual citizenship in Italy and the United States.

In 1948 it was discovered in Hamburger's laboratory that a variety of mouse tumour spurred nerve growth when implanted into chick embryos. Levi-Montalcini and Hamburger traced the effect to a substance in the tumour that they named nerve-growth factor (NGF). Levi-Montalcini further showed that the tumour caused similar cell growth in a nerve-tissue culture kept alive in the laboratory, and Stanley Cohen, who by then had joined her at Washington University, was able to isolate the NGF from the tumour. NGF was the first of many cell-growth factors to be found in the bodies of animals. It plays an important role in the growth of nerve cells and fibres in the peripheral nervous system.

Levi-Montalcini established the Institute of Cell Biology in Rome in 1962 and thereafter divided her time between the institute and Washington University. In 1987 she was awarded the National Medal of Science, and an autobiographical work, *In Praise of Imperfection,* was published in 1988. In 2001 Italian Prime Minister Carlo Azeglio Ciampi appointed Levi-Montalcini senator for life for her outstanding contributions to science.

VIRGINIA APGAR

(born June 7, 1909, Westfield, N.J., U.S.–died Aug. 7, 1974, New York, N.Y.)

Virginia Apgar was an American physician, anesthesiologist, and medical researcher who developed the Apgar Score System, a method of evaluating an infant shortly after birth to assess its well-being and to determine if any immediate medical intervention is required.

Apgar graduated from Mount Holyoke College in 1929 and from the Columbia University College of Physicians and Surgeons in 1933. After an internship at

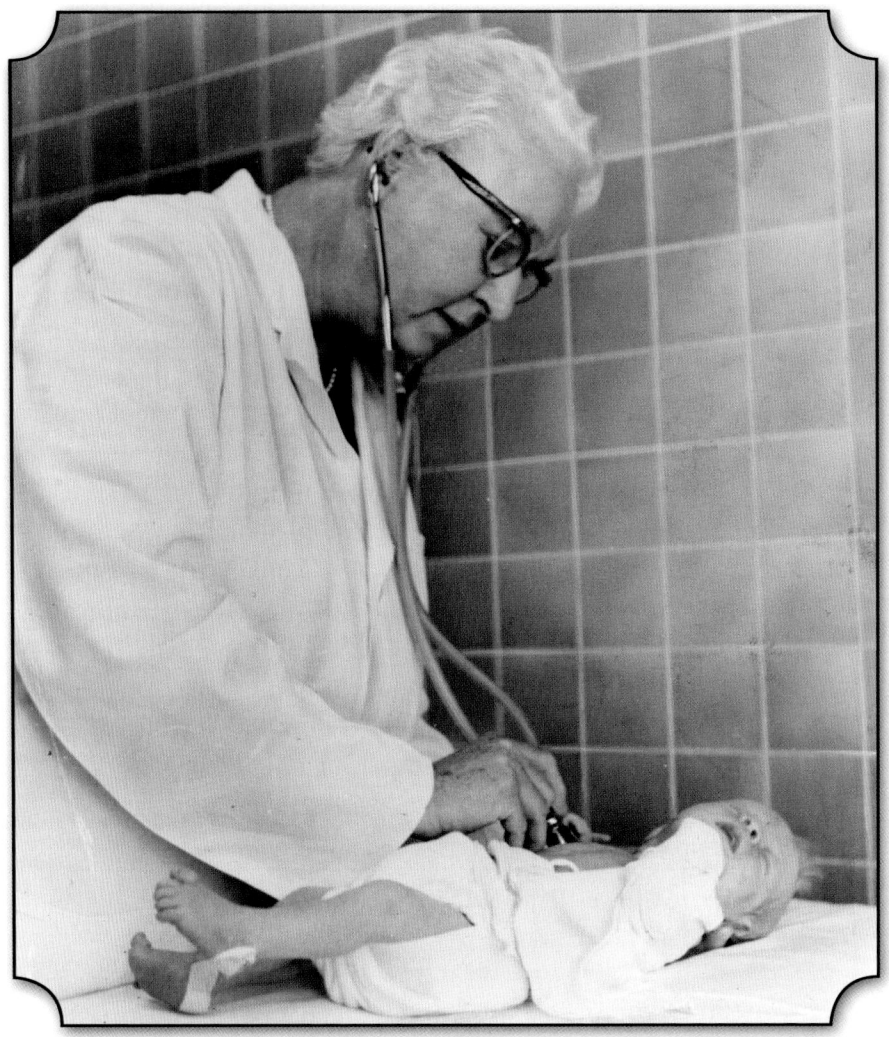

Virginia Apgar examines a baby in 1966.

Presbyterian Hospital, New York City, she held residencies in the relatively new specialty of anesthesiology at the University of Wisconsin and then at Bellevue Hospital, New York City, in 1935–37. In 1937 she became the first female board-certified anesthesiologist. The first professor of anesthesiology at the College of Physicians and Surgeons (1949–59), she was also the first female physician to attain the rank of full professor there. Additionally, from 1938 she was director of the department of anesthesiology at Columbia-Presbyterian Medical Center.

An interest in obstetric procedure, and particularly in the treatment of the newborn, led her to develop a simple system for quickly evaluating the condition and viability of newly delivered infants. As finally presented in 1952, the Apgar Score System relies on five simple observations to be made by delivery room personnel (nurses or interns) of the infant within one minute of birth and—depending on the results of the first observation—periodically thereafter. The Apgar Score System soon came into general use throughout the United States and was adopted by several other countries.

Five signs are assessed in the Apgar Score System: heart rate, respiratory effort, muscle tone, reflex irritability, and skin colour. Medical students memorize these signs by using the mnemonic of Apgar's name: *a*ppearance, *p*ulse, *g*rimace, *a*ctivity, and *r*espiration. A score of 0, 1, or 2 is assigned to each component. Usually, the higher the total score, with 10 being the maximum, the better the infant's condition. If the infant's total score is less than 7, it is reevaluated every 5 minutes until 20 minutes have passed or until two successive scores of 7 or greater are obtained.

According to some researchers, the one- and five-minute Apgar scores are of limited use in predicting the degree of asphyxia (lack of oxygen or excess of carbon dioxide) or the consequences of any neurological involvement. Apgar scores taken at 10 or 15 minutes may be more successful indicators of an infant's later neurological deficit.

In 1959 Apgar left Columbia and took a degree in public health from Johns Hopkins University. She headed the division of congenital malformations at the National Foundation-March of Dimes from 1959–67. She was promoted to director of basic research at the National Foundation (1967–72), and she later became senior vice president for medical affairs (1973–74). She cowrote the book *Is My Baby All Right?* (1972) with Joan Beck.

PAUL MAURICE ZOLL
(born July 15, 1911, Boston, Mass.–died Jan. 5, 1999, Chestnut Hill, near Boston)

Paul Maurice Zoll conducted pioneering research that led to the development of the cardiac defibrillator, improved pacemakers, and continuous heart-rhythm monitoring devices. Following his graduation from Harvard College (B.A., 1932) and Harvard Medical School (M.D., 1936), Zoll was made a research fellow (1939) in cardiology at Beth Israel Hospital, Boston, working under physicians Monroe Schlesinger and Herman Blumgart. During World War II he was stationed in Great Britain as a U.S. Army physician. In that capacity he observed numerous open-heart surgeries performed by Dwight Harken, and he noted with interest the manner in which the heart responded reflexively to the slightest touch.

After the war he became involved in attempts to regulate the heartbeat and treat myocardial infarctions (heart attacks). At the time, emergency cardiac resuscitation involved cutting patients' chests open and squeezing the heart by hand. Zoll experimented with closed-chest electrical cardiac stimulation, and in 1952 he restarted the hearts of two patients at Beth Israel Hospital. Researchers worldwide were soon racing to enhance defibrillator designs, which later became standard issue in emergency rooms, ambulances, and airplanes. Acceptance from within the medical community was not universal or immediate, however; many questioned whether such "artificial" methods were ethical if not altogether blasphemous.

Zoll's efforts were later concentrated on improving cardiac pacemakers, which were massive, inefficient external machines that often caused great pain to their users. His new designs were the forerunners of the miniaturized permanent pacemakers currently implanted in hundreds of thousands of patients each year. Zoll also worked to improve electrocardiographic monitoring devices. In the 1980s he founded ZOLL Medical Corp., which developed and marketed new defibrillator designs. Despite his numerous contributions to medical technology, Zoll received only limited recognition until 1973, when he was awarded the Albert Lasker Clinical Medical Research Award.

JONAS SALK

(born Oct. 28, 1914, New York, N.Y., U.S.–died June 23, 1995, La Jolla, Calif.)

Jonas Salk (in full Jonas Edward Salk) was an American physician and medical researcher who developed the first safe and effective vaccine for polio.

Salk received an M.D. in 1939 from New York University College of Medicine, where he worked with Thomas Francis, Jr., who was conducting killed-virus immunology studies. Salk joined Francis in 1942 at the University of Michigan School of Public Health and became part of a group that was working to develop an immunization against influenza.

In 1947 Salk became associate professor of bacteriology and head of the Virus Research Laboratory at the University of Pittsburgh School of Medicine. At Pittsburgh he began research on polio, an acute viral infectious disease of the nervous system that usually begins with general symptoms such as fever and headache and is sometimes followed by a more serious and permanent paralysis of muscles in one or more limbs, the throat, or the chest. In the mid-20th century hundreds of thousands of children were struck by the disease every year. Working with scientists from other universities in a program to classify the various strains of poliovirus, Salk corroborated other studies in identifying three separate strains. He then demonstrated that killed virus of each of the three, although incapable of producing the disease, could induce antibody formation in monkeys.

In 1952 he conducted field tests of his killed-virus vaccine, first on children who had recovered from polio and then on subjects who had not had the disease; both tests were successful in that the children's antibody levels rose significantly and no subjects contracted polio from the vaccine. His findings were published the following year. In 1954 Francis conducted a mass field trial, and the vaccine, injected by needle, was found to safely reduce the incidence of polio. On April 12, 1955, the vaccine was released for use in the United States. In the following years the incidence of polio in the United States fell from 18 cases per 100,000 people to less than 2 per 100,000. In the 1960s a second type of polio vaccine, known as oral poliovirus vaccine (OPV) or Sabin vaccine—named for its inventor, American physician and microbiologist Albert Sabin—was developed. OPV contains live attenuated (weakened) virus and is given orally.

Salk served successively as professor of bacteriology, preventive medicine, and experimental medicine at Pittsburgh, and in 1963 he became fellow and director of the Institute for Biological Studies in San Diego, Calif., later called the Salk Institute. Among his many honours was the Presidential Medal of Freedom, awarded in 1977.

FRANCIS HARRY COMPTON CRICK
(born June 8, 1916, Northampton, Northamptonshire, England–died July 28, 2004, San Diego, Calif., U.S.)

Francis Crick was a British biophysicist, who, with James Watson and Maurice Wilkins, received the 1962 Nobel Prize for Physiology or Medicine for their determination of the molecular structure of deoxyribonucleic acid (DNA), the chemical substance ultimately responsible for hereditary control of life functions. This accomplishment became a cornerstone of genetics and was widely regarded as one of the most important discoveries of 20th-century biology.

During World War II, Crick interrupted his education to work as a physicist in the development of magnetic mines for use in naval warfare, but afterward he turned to biology at the Strangeways Research Laboratory, University of Cambridge (1947). Interested in pioneering efforts to determine the three-dimensional structures of large molecules found in living organisms, he transferred to the university's Medical Research Council Unit at the Cavendish Laboratories in 1949.

In 1951, when the American biologist James Watson arrived at the laboratory, it was known that the mysterious nucleic acids, especially DNA, played a central role in the hereditary determination of the structure and function of each cell. Watson convinced Crick that knowledge of DNA's three-dimensional structure would make its hereditary role apparent. Using the X-ray diffraction studies of DNA done by Wilkins and X-ray diffraction pictures produced by Rosalind Franklin, Watson and Crick were able to construct a molecular model consistent with the known physical and chemical properties of DNA. The model consisted of two intertwined helical (spiral) strands of sugar-phosphate, bridged horizontally by flat organic bases. Watson and Crick theorized that if the strands were separated, each would serve as a template (pattern) for the formation, from small molecules in the cell, of a new sister strand identical to its former partner. This copying process explained replication of the gene and, eventually, the chromosome, known to occur in dividing cells. Their model also indicated that the sequence of bases along the DNA molecule spells some kind of code "read" by a cellular mechanism that translates it into the specific proteins responsible for a cell's particular structure and function.

By 1961 Crick had evidence to show that each group of three bases (a codon) on a single DNA strand designates the position of a specific amino acid on the backbone of a protein molecule. He also helped to determine which codons code for each of the 20 amino acids normally found in protein and thus helped clarify the way in which the cell eventually uses the DNA "message" to build proteins. From 1977 until his death, Crick held the position of distinguished professor at the Salk Institute for Biological Studies in San Diego, Calif., where he conducted research on the neurological basis of consciousness. His book *Of Molecules and Men* (1966) discusses the implications of the revolution in molecular biology. *What Mad Pursuit: A Personal View of*

Scientific Discovery was published in 1988. In 1991 Crick received the Order of Merit.

ADRIAN KANTROWITZ
(born Oct. 4, 1918, New York, N.Y., U.S.–died Nov. 14, 2008, Ann Arbor, Mich.)

Adrian Kantrowitz was a pioneer in the development of mechanical hearts and other devices to improve heart function. In 1967 he performed the first human heart transplant in the United States at Maimonides Medical Center in New York City. Kantrowitz was an adjunct surgeon (1951–55) at Montefiore (N.Y.) Hospital and served (1955–70) in various surgical posts at Maimonides. His innovations in human heart-related technology began early in his medical career.

In 1951 he made the first film to show the inside of a beating human heart. He introduced an improved heart-lung machine in 1958, a pacemaker small enough to implant in 1962, and a balloon pump for short-term use after surgery in 1967. Kantrowitz transplanted a human heart into an infant on Dec. 6, 1967, just three days after South African surgeon Christiaan Barnard performed the world's first human heart transplant. Kantrowitz moved to Detroit, where he chaired the department of surgery (1970–75) and the department of cardiovascular surgery (1975–83) at Sinai Hospital. He also served as professor of surgery at Wayne State University School of Medicine in Detroit. In 1983 he and his wife, Jean Rosensaft Kantrowitz, founded LVAD Technology, a research firm that focused on developing new cardiovascular devices. The American Society of Artificial Internal Organs presented Kantrowitz with a lifetime achievement award in 2001.

JOSEPH E. MURRAY

(born April 1, 1919, Milford, Mass.s, U.S.–died Nov. 26, 2012, Boston, Mass.)

Joseph E. Muray (in full Joseph Edward Murray) was an American surgeon who in 1990 was cowinner (with E. Donnall Thomas) of the Nobel Prize for Physiology or Medicine for his work in lifesaving organ- and tissue-transplant techniques.

Murray received a bachelor of arts degree (1940) from Holy Cross College, Worcester, Mass., and a medical degree (1943) from Harvard Medical School, Cambridge, Mass. He completed his surgical residency at Peter Bent Brigham Hospital (later Brigham and Women's Hospital), Boston, where he began his prize-winning research. From 1964 to 1986 he served as chief plastic surgeon at Brigham, and from 1972 to 1985 he was chief plastic surgeon at Children's Hospital Medical Center, Boston. He also became professor of surgery at Harvard Medical School in 1970; he retired as professor emeritus in 1986.

While grafting skin on wounded soldiers during World War II, Murray observed that grafts were compatible only between identical twins. Thinking that such might be the case for transplanted internal organs as well, he experimented with kidney transplants in dogs. In 1954 he performed a kidney transplant for an individual whose genetically identical twin volunteered to donate a kidney; the recipient survived for several years. Murray continued to search for ways of suppressing a patient's immune system to keep it from rejecting genetically foreign parts. With the use of immunosuppressive drugs, in 1962 he performed the first successful kidney transplant using a kidney from a donor unrelated to his patient. Eventually he was able to successfully transplant a kidney from a cadaver.

In 2001 Murray published an autobiography, *Surgery of the Soul: Reflections on a Curious Career*; the book was praised by physicians and others in the medical community for its insight into medical practice.

ROSALIND FRANKLIN
(born July 25, 1920, London, England–died April 16, 1958, London)

Rosalind Franklin (in full Rosalind Elsie Franklin) was a British scientist who contributed to the discovery of the molecular structure of DNA, a constituent of chromosomes that serves to encode genetic information.

Franklin attended St. Paul's Girls' School before studying physical chemistry at Newnham College, Cambridge. After graduating in 1941, she received a fellowship to conduct research in physical chemistry at Cambridge. But the advance of World War II changed her course of action: not only did she serve as a London air raid warden, but in 1942 she gave up her fellowship in order to work for the British Coal Utilisation Research Association, where she investigated the physical chemistry of carbon and coal for the war effort.

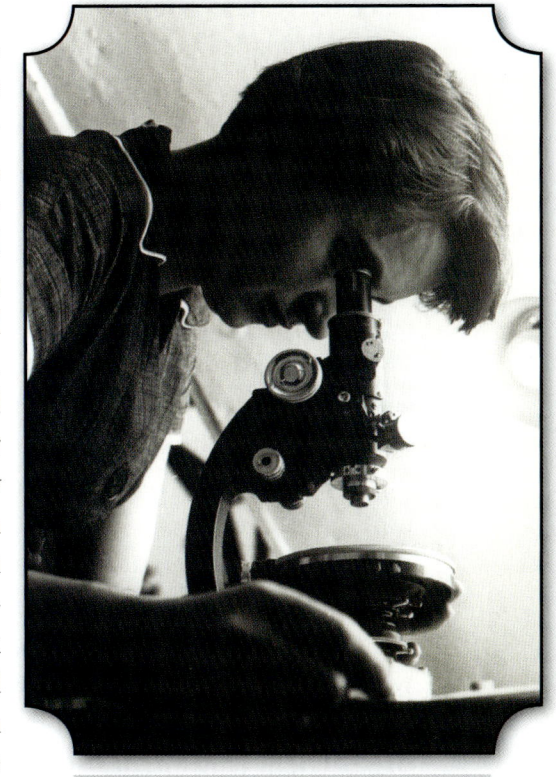

Although she died before the implications of her work were recognized, Rosalind Franklin's research was essential to the discovery of the structure of DNA.

Nevertheless, she was able to use this research for her doctoral thesis, and in 1945 she received a doctorate from Cambridge. From 1947 to 1950 she worked with Jacques Méring at the State Chemical Laboratory in Paris, studying X-ray diffraction technology. That work led to her research on the structural changes caused by the formation of graphite in heated carbons—work that proved valuable for the coking industry.

In 1951 Franklin joined the Biophysical Laboratory at King's College, London, as a research fellow. There she applied X-ray diffraction methods to the study of DNA. When she began her research at King's College, very little was known about the chemical makeup or structure of DNA. However, she soon discovered the density of DNA and, more importantly, established that the molecule existed in a helical conformation. Her work to make clearer X-ray patterns of DNA molecules laid the foundation for James Watson and Francis Crick to suggest in 1953 that the structure of DNA is a double-helix polymer, a spiral z consisting of two DNA strands wound around each other.

From 1953 to 1958 Franklin worked in the Crystallography Laboratory at Birkbeck College, London. While there she completed her work on coals and on DNA and began a project on the molecular structure of the tobacco mosaic virus. She collaborated on studies showing that the ribonucleic acid (RNA) in that virus was embedded in its protein rather than in its central cavity and that this RNA was a single-strand helix, rather than the double helix found in the DNA of bacterial viruses and higher organisms. Franklin's involvement in cutting-edge DNA research was halted by her untimely death from cancer in 1958.

DENTON A. COOLEY
(born Aug. 22, 1920, Houston, Tex., U.S.)

Denton A. Cooley (in full Denton Arthur Cooley) is an American surgeon and educator chiefly noted for heart-transplant operations. He was also the first to implant an artificial heart in a human. In April 1969 Cooley observed that the heart of a 47-year-old patient would not function adequately after he removed a section of diseased heart muscle. He implanted a mechanical heart made of silicone, which served as a substitute organ for 65 hours until a heart from a human donor was inserted to replace it. Nevertheless, the patient died 38 hours after the second operation because of pneumonia and kidney failure.

Cooley received an M.D. degree from Johns Hopkins University, Baltimore (1944), and joined the medical faculty of Baylor University College of Medicine, Houston, in 1954. In 1969 he left Baylor to found the Texas Heart Institute, of which he became president and surgeon in chief, and from 1975 he served also as professor of clinical surgery at the University of Texas Medical School in Houston. In 1998 Cooley received the National Medal of Technology, the highest honour for technological innovation.

ROSALYN S. YALOW
(born July 19, 1921, New York, N.Y., U.S.–died May 30, 2011, New York)

Rosalyn S. Yalow (in full Rosalyn Sussman Yalow) was an American medical physicist and joint recipient (with Andrew V. Schally and Roger Guillemin) of the 1977 Nobel Prize for Physiology or Medicine, awarded for her development of radioimmunoassay (RIA), an extremely sensitive technique for measuring minute quantities of biologically active substances.

Yalow graduated with honours from Hunter College of the City University of New York in 1941 and four years later received her Ph.D. in physics from the University of Illinois. From 1946 to 1950 she lectured on physics at Hunter, and in 1947 she became a consultant in nuclear physics to the Bronx Veterans Administration Hospital, where from 1950 to 1970 she was physicist and assistant chief of the radioisotope service.

With a colleague, the American physician Solomon A. Berson, Yalow began using radioactive isotopes to examine and diagnose various disease conditions. Yalow and Berson's investigations into the mechanism underlying type II diabetes led to their development of RIA. In the 1950s it was known that individuals treated with injections of animal insulin developed resistance to the hormone and so required greater amounts of it to offset the effects of the disease; however, a satisfactory explanation for this phenomenon had not been put forth. Yalow and Berson theorized that the foreign insulin stimulated the production of antibodies, which became bound to the insulin and prevented the hormone from entering cells and carrying out its function of metabolizing glucose. In order to prove their hypothesis to a skeptical scientific community, the researchers combined techniques from immunology and radioisotope tracing to measure minute amounts of these antibodies, and the RIA was born. It was soon apparent that this method could be used to measure hundreds of other biologically active substances, such as viruses, drugs, and other proteins. This made possible such practical applications as the screening of blood in blood banks for hepatitis virus and the determination of effective dosage levels of drugs and antibiotics.

In 1970 Yalow was appointed chief of the laboratory later renamed the Nuclear Medical Service at the Veterans Administration Hospital. In 1976 she was the first female recipient of the Albert Lasker Basic Medical Research Award. Yalow became a distinguished professor at large at the Albert Einstein College of Medicine at Yeshiva University in 1979 and left in 1985 to accept the position of Solomon A. Berson Distinguished Professor at Large at the Mount Sinai School of Medicine. She was awarded the National Medal of Science in 1988.

CHRISTIAAN BARNARD

(born Nov. 8, 1922, Beaufort West, South Africa–died Sept. 2, 2001, Paphos, Cyprus)

Christiaan Barnard (in full Christiaan Neethling Barnard) was a South African surgeon who performed the first transplant of a heart from one human to another (1967); the first "piggyback" heart transplant, in which a second heart was inserted in order to aid the patient's own weak one (1974); the first transplantation of an animal's heart into a human, again to assist the patient's heart and give it time to heal (1977); and the first heart-lung transplant (1981).

Barnard graduated from the University of Cape Town in 1946, spent some time in private practice, and then returned to the university to conduct research. He earned his M.D. degree in 1953. As a resident surgeon at Groote Schuur Hospital, Cape Town (1953–56), Barnard was the first to show that intestinal atresia, a congenital gap in the small intestine, is caused by an insufficient blood supply to the fetus during pregnancy. This discovery led to the development of a surgical procedure to correct the formerly fatal defect. After completing doctoral studies at the University of Minnesota (1956–58), he returned to the hospital as senior cardiothoracic surgeon, bringing a U.S. government-donated heart-lung machine with him. Barnard introduced open-heart surgery to South Africa and developed a new design for artificial heart valves.

At Groote Schuur he formed one of the world's finest heart-surgery units, where he had especially good results with valve surgery and with correcting children's congenital cardiac problems and where he also began experimenting with heart transplantation, generally in dogs. On Dec. 3, 1967, Barnard led a team of 20 surgeons in replacing the heart of Louis Washkansky, an incurably ill South African grocer, with a heart taken from a fatally injured accident victim. Although the transplant itself was successful, Washkansky died 18 days later from double pneumonia, contracted after destruction of his body's immunity mechanism by drugs administered to suppress rejection of the new heart as a foreign protein. His second patient lived more than 19 months. More experience and the development of better antirejection drugs eventually made heart transplant surgery standard, and some 100,000 such operations had been performed by the time Barnard died in late 2001.

His early transplants were daring and controversial, in part because they set a precedent for the consideration of brain death as acceptable for the harvesting of organs for transplant and in part because he flouted the racial barriers of apartheid. They also gained the handsome and charismatic doctor instant fame both professionally and socially, and he became an international celebrity and member of the jet set.

Barnard's later transplant operations were increasingly successful; by the late 1970s a number of his patients had survived for several years. Barnard served as the head of the cardiac unit at Groote Schuur Hospital until 1983, at which time he retired from active surgical practice. He thereafter included conducting research in Oklahoma, running his farm in South Africa, and writing a weekly newspaper column among his activities. In addition to the autobiography *One Life* (1969; with Curtis Bill Pepper)—whose royalties were donated to the Chris Barnard Foundation, which supported research and made it possible for children from all over the world to travel to South Africa for heart surgery—Barnard also wrote papers for scholarly journals and a number of other books, including another autobiography, *The Second Life* (1993), such works on health topics as *Heart Attack: You Don't Have to Die* (1971), *The Arthritis Handbook* (1984), and *50 Ways to a Healthy Heart* (2001), and several novels.

STANLEY COHEN
(born Nov. 17, 1922, Brooklyn, New York, N.Y., U.S.)

Stanley Cohen is an American biochemist who, with Rita Levi-Montalcini, shared the 1986 Nobel Prize for Physiology or Medicine for his researches on substances produced in the body that influence the development of nerve and skin tissues.

Cohen was educated at Brooklyn College (B.A., 1943), Oberlin College (M.A., 1945), and at the University of Michigan, where he received a Ph.D. in biochemistry in 1948. He joined Levi-Montalcini at Washington University, St. Louis, Mo., as a researcher in 1952. His training as a biochemist enabled him to help isolate nerve growth factor, a natural substance that Levi-Montalcini had found stimulated the growth of nerve cells and fibres. Cohen found another cell growth factor in the chemical extracts that contained the nerve growth factor. He discovered that this substance caused the eyes of newborn mice to open and their teeth to erupt several days sooner than normal. Cohen termed this substance epidermal growth factor (EGF), and he went on to purify it and completely analyze its chemistry. He and his coworkers found that EGF influences a great range of developmental events in the body. He also discovered the mechanisms by which EGF is taken into and acts upon individual cells.

Cohen conducted his research at Washington University until 1959, upon which he moved to Vanderbilt University, Nashville, Tenn., becoming professor of biochemistry there in 1967. Cohen later received an Albert Lasker Basic Medical Research Award (1986) and was inducted into the National Institute of Child Health and Human Development Hall of Honor (2007).

ALEXANDER GORDON BEARN

(born March 29, 1923, Cheam, Surrey, England–died May 15, 2009, Philadelphia, Pa., U.S.)

Alexander Gordon Bearn was a British-born American physician and geneticist who discovered the hereditary nature of Wilson disease and established the basis for diagnostic tests and novel forms of treatment for the disease. Bearn's work, which provided an important model for the identification, diagnosis, and treatment of other genetic diseases, served to bridge the gap between genetics and medicine that existed in the 1950s.

EDUCATION AND CAREER AT ROCKEFELLER

Bearn was one of three children, and his father worked for the Ministry of Health in Britain. Bearn received a Bachelor of Medicine degree in 1946 from King's College School of Medicine and Dentistry, University of London. He continued his doctoral studies there, eventually receiving a doctorate of medicine degree in 1950. The following year he left England to take a position as an assistant professor at the Rockefeller Institute for Medical Research (now Rockefeller University) in New York City. There Bearn became interested in the genetic mutations underlying rare metabolic diseases and eventually narrowed his research, focusing on Wilson disease. Although diseases caused by hereditary defects had been described in the early 20th century, they were not understood well enough to facilitate their diagnosis or to encourage the development of improved treatments. Thus, when Bearn began investigating Wilson disease, genetics was of little consequence to medicine. In 1957 Bearn established one of the first human genetics laboratories in the United States at Rockefeller, and in 1964 he became a professor of medicine there.

Research on Wilson Disease

Wilson disease was described as progressive lenticular degeneration in 1912 by American-born British neurologist Samuel A.K. Wilson. Wilson's autopsies of affected patients revealed cirrhosis of the liver and degeneration of the lenticular nucleus, a part of the brain located within the basal ganglia. In the following decades, it was found that the liver and brain served as sites for the accumulation of copper, which was discovered to be the underlying pathological feature of the disease. Although Wilson and others found that the disease occurred within families, it was not recognized as a hereditary condition. In fact, it was not until the 1950s, when Bearn studied families affected by Wilson disease and found that it was inherited in an autosomal recessive fashion, that the hereditary nature of the condition was realized. The recessive inheritance of Wilson disease meant that two copies (one from each parent) of the abnormal gene were required to cause the disease.

Bearn proposed that the specific genetic defect of Wilson disease, which was unknown then, somehow altered the transport of copper into and out of cells. Bearn suggested that a serum protein called ceruloplasmin, which transports copper through the blood and is present in abnormally low levels in Wilson disease patients, could be used as a diagnostic measure for the disease. In addition, decreased serum levels and decreased urinary excretion of copper also could serve as measures for diagnosis. For the treatment of Wilson disease, Bearn promoted the use of penicillamine, a chelating agent that lowers tissue concentrations of copper by drawing the element out of cells and facilitating its excretion in the urine. Bearn also encouraged patients to avoid eating foods that are high in copper.

LATER CAREER

In 1966 Bearn was appointed chairman of the department of medicine at Cornell University Medical College. He subsequently established a human genetics laboratory there and became physician in chief at New York Hospital (now New York–Presbyterian Hospital). While at Cornell, Bearn helped initiate a joint M.D./Ph.D. program between Cornell and Rockefeller. In 1970 Bearn joined Rockefeller's board of trustees, and the following year he became president of the American Society of Human Genetics. In 1972 he was elected a member of the American Philosophical Society, a prestigious organization founded by Benjamin Franklin in 1743. Bearn later served as vice president (1990–96) and as executive officer (1997–2002) of the society and was elected a member of the National Academy of Science. From 1979 to 1988 Bearn served as senior vice president for medical and scientific affairs for the pharmaceutical company Merck & Co., Inc.

Following his retirement from Cornell in 1988, Bearn wrote *Sir Archibald Garrod and the Individuality of Man* (1993), which explores the life and discoveries of Garrod, who was a British physician and geneticist known for his investigations into inherited metabolic diseases in the early 1900s. Bearn later wrote two other biographies, *Sir Clifford Allbutt: Scholar and Physician* (2007) and *Sir Francis Richard Fraser: A Canny Scot Shapes British Medicine* (2008).

ROGER CHARLES LOUIS GUILLEMIN
(born Jan. 11, 1924, Dijon, France)

French-born American Roger Charles Louis Guillemin is a physiologist whose research into the hormones produced by the hypothalamus gland resulted in his being awarded a share (along with Andrew Schally and Rosalyn Yalow) of the Nobel Prize for Physiology or Medicine in 1977.

Guillemin was educated at the universities of Dijon, Lyon, and Montreal. He taught at the Baylor College of Medicine in Houston, Texas, from 1953 to 1970, except for the years 1960–63, when he was on the faculty of the Collège de France in Paris. From 1970 he was a resident fellow and research professor at the Salk Institute for Biological Studies in La Jolla, Calif. Guillemin became a U.S. citizen in 1963.

Guillemin proved the hypothesis that the hypothalamus releases hormones that regulate the pituitary gland. Among the hypothalamic hormones that he and his colleagues discovered, isolated, analyzed, or synthesized were TRH (thyrotropin-releasing hormone), which regulates thyroid activity; GHRH (growth hormone-releasing hormone), which causes the pituitary to release gonadotropin; and somatostatin, which regulates the activities of the pituitary gland and the pancreas. Guillemin also discovered an important class of proteins called endorphins that are involved in the perception of pain.

BARUCH S. BLUMBERG
(born July 28, 1925, Brooklyn, N.Y., U.S.–died April 5, 2011, Moffett Field, near Mountain View, Calif.)

Baruch S. Blumberg (in full Baruch Samuel Blumberg) was an American research physician whose discovery of an antigen that provokes antibody response against hepatitis B led to the development by other researchers of a successful vaccine against the disease. He shared the Nobel Prize for Physiology or Medicine in 1976 with D. Carleton Gajdusek for their work on the origins and spread of infectious viral diseases.

Blumberg received an M.D. degree from Columbia University's College of Physicians and Surgeons in 1951 and a Ph.D. degree in biochemistry from the University of Oxford in 1957. In 1960 he became chief of the Geographic Medicine and Genetics Section of the U.S. National Institutes of Health, Bethesda, Md. In 1964 he was appointed associate director for clinical research at the Institute for Cancer Research (later named the Fox Chase Cancer Center) in Philadelphia. He also served as professor of medicine, human genetics, and anthropology at the University of Pennsylvania. In 1989 Blumberg became the first Fox Chase Distinguished Scientist, and he returned to Oxford to become master of Balliol College, a position that he held until 1994. Upon his return to the United States, he continued to teach as professor of medicine and anthropology at the University of Pennsylvania. From 1999 to 2002 Blumberg served as director of the National Aeronautics and Space Administration (NASA)

Astrobiology Institute, where he embarked on investigations into the possibility of life on other planets. He held several different positions while at NASA, where he remained until 2004. The following year he was elected president of the American Philosophical Society; he held the post until his death.

In the early 1960s Blumberg was examining blood samples from widely diverse populations in an attempt to determine why the members of different ethnic and national groups vary widely in their responses and susceptibility to disease. In 1963 he discovered in the blood serum of an Australian Aborigine an antigen that he later (1967) determined to be part of a virus that causes hepatitis B, the most-severe form of hepatitis. The discovery of that so-called Australian antigen, which causes the body to produce antibody responses to the virus, made it possible to screen blood donors for possible hepatitis B transmission. Further research indicated that the body's development of an antibody against the Australian antigen was protective against further infection with the virus itself. In 1982 a safe and effective vaccine utilizing the Australian antigen was made commercially available in the United States. Blumberg's book on his Nobel Prize-winning work, *Hepatitis B: The Hunt for a Killer Virus*, was published in 2002.

ANDREW V. SCHALLY

(born Nov. 30, 1926, Wilno, Poland [now Vilnius, Lithuania])

Andrew V. Schally (in full Andrew Victor Schally) is a Polish-born American endocrinologist and corecipient, with Roger Guillemin and Rosalyn Yalow, of the 1977 Nobel Prize for Physiology or Medicine. He was noted for isolating and synthesizing three hormones that are produced by the region of the brain known as the hypothalamus; these hormones control the activities of other hormone-producing glands.

Schally fled Poland with his family in 1939. He attended the University of London and worked for three years at the National Institute for Medical Research in London before traveling to Montreal to enter McGill University. He graduated in 1955 and two years later took a Ph.D. in biochemistry. From 1957 to 1962 he was associated with Baylor University in Houston, Texas, and in 1962 he became a U.S. citizen. That same year Schally was made chief of endocrine and polypeptide laboratories at the Veterans Administration (VA) Medical Center in New Orleans, La. At the same time he joined the medical faculty of the Tulane University School of Medicine, becoming a professor in 1967. He became senior medical investigator with the VA in 1973.

Among Schally's chief accomplishments were the synthesis of TRH (thyrotropin-releasing hormone), the isolation and synthesis of LHRH (luteinizing hormone-releasing hormone), and studies of the action of the peptide somatostatin. His research helped elucidate pathways of hormone regulation in males and females and contributed to the development of fertility treatments and contraceptives. In 1975 Schally and Guillemin received the Albert Lasker Basic Medical Research Award.

JAMES DEWEY WATSON
(born April 6, 1928, Chicago, Ill., U.S.)

James Dewey Watson is an American geneticist and biophysicist who played a crucial role in the discovery of the molecular structure of DNA, the substance that is the basis of heredity. For this accomplishment he was awarded the 1962 Nobel Prize for Physiology or Medicine with Francis Crick and Maurice Wilkins.

Watson enrolled at the University of Chicago when only 15 and graduated in 1947. From his virus research at Indiana University (Ph.D., 1950), and from the experiments of Canadian-born American bacteriologist Oswald Avery, which proved that DNA affects hereditary traits, Watson became convinced that the gene could be understood only after something was known about nucleic acid molecules. He learned that scientists working in the Cavendish Laboratory at the University of Cambridge were using photographic patterns made by X-rays that had been shot through protein crystals to study the structure of protein molecules.

After working at the University of Copenhagen, where he first determined to investigate DNA, he did research at the Cavendish Laboratory (1951–53). There Watson learned X-ray diffraction techniques and worked with Crick on the problem of DNA structure. In 1952 he determined the structure of the protein coat surrounding the tobacco mosaic virus but made no dramatic progress with DNA. Suddenly, in the spring of 1953, Watson saw that the essential DNA components—four organic bases—must be linked in definite pairs. This discovery was the key factor that enabled Watson and Crick to formulate a molecular model for DNA—a double helix, which can be likened to a spiraling staircase or a twisting ladder. The DNA double helix consists of two intertwined sugar-phosphate chains, with the flat base pairs forming the steps between them. Watson and Crick's model also shows how the DNA molecule could duplicate itself. Thus, it became known how genes, and eventually chromosomes, duplicate themselves. Watson and Crick published their epochal discovery in two papers in the British journal *Nature* in April–May 1953. Their research answered one of the fundamental questions in genetics.

Watson subsequently taught at Harvard University

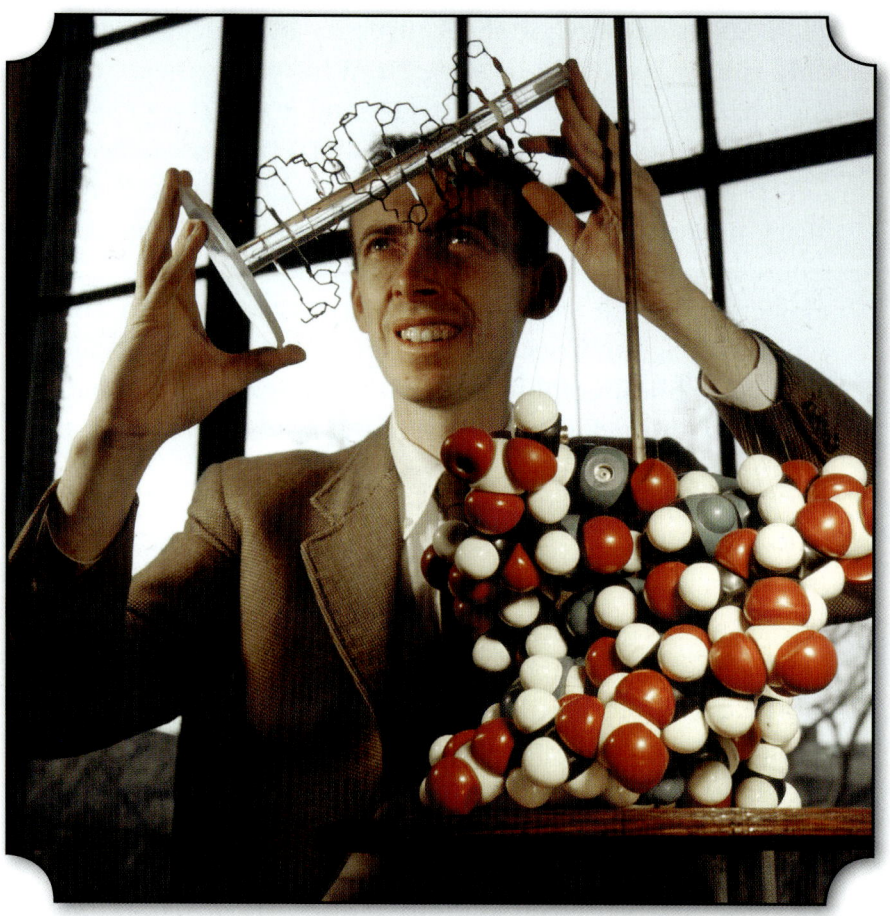

James Watson examines a model of DNA. Building on the work of Rosalind Franklin, he and Francis Crick discovered the double helix structure of DNA.

(1955–76), where he served as professor of biology (1961–76). He conducted research on the role of nucleic acids in the synthesis of proteins. In 1965 he published *Molecular Biology of the Gene,* one of the most extensively used modern biology texts. He later wrote *The Double Helix* (1968), an informal, personal account of the DNA discovery and the roles of the people involved in it, which aroused some controversy. In 1968 Watson assumed the leadership of the Laboratory of Quantitative Biology at Cold Spring Harbor, Long Island, N.Y., and made it a world centre for research in molecular biology. He concentrated its efforts on cancer research. In 1981 his *The DNA Story* (written with John Tooze) was published. From 1988 to 1992 at the National Institutes of Health, Watson helped direct the Human Genome Project, a project to map and decipher all the genes in the human chromosomes, but he eventually resigned because of alleged conflicts of interest involving his investments in private biotechnology companies.

In early 2007 Watson's own genome was sequenced and made publicly available on the Internet. He was the second person in history to have a personal genome sequenced in its entirety. In October of the same year, he sparked controversy by making a public statement referring to the idea that the intelligence of Africans might not be the same as that of other peoples and that intellectual differences between geographically separated peoples might arise over time as a result of genetic divergence. Watson's remarks were immediately denounced as racist. Though he denied this charge, he resigned from his position at Cold Spring Harbor and formally announced his retirement less than two weeks later.

LUC MONTAGNIER
(born Aug. 18, 1932, Chabris, France)

Luc Montagnier is a French research scientist who received, with Harald zur Hausen and Francoise Barré-Sinoussi, the 2008 Nobel Prize for Physiology or Medicine. Montagnier and Barré-Sinoussi shared half the prize for their work in identifying the human immunodeficiency virus (HIV), the cause of acquired immunodeficiency syndrome (AIDS).

Montagnier was educated at the Universities of Poitiers and Paris, earning degrees in science (1953) and medicine (1960). He began his career as a research scientist in 1955 and joined the Pasteur Institute in Paris in 1972. In 1993 he established the World Foundation for AIDS Research and Prevention, and he later accepted an endowed chair at Queens College, New York City, where he headed (1998–2001) the Center for Molecular and Cellular Biology. He returned to the Pasteur Institute in 2001 as professor emeritus. Montagnier also served as president of the Administrative Council of the European Federation for AIDS Research.

In the early 1980s Montagnier, working at the Pasteur Institute with a team that included Barré-Sinoussi, identified the retrovirus that eventually became known as HIV. In the ensuing years there was much controversy over who first isolated the virus, Montagnier or American scientist Robert Gallo, and in 1987 the U.S. and French governments agreed to share credit for the discovery. Subsequently, however, Montagnier's team was generally acknowledged as having first identified the virus.

OLIVER SACKS

(born July 9, 1933, London, England–Aug. 30, 2015, New York, N.Y., U.S.)

Oliver Sacks (in full Oliver Wolf Sacks) was a British neurologist and writer who won acclaim for his sympathetic case histories of patients with unusual neurological disorders.

Sacks spent most of his childhood in London, though his parents, both general practitioners trained as neurologists, sent him to a boarding school for four years during

World War II to escape the air raids then strafing the city. Sacks attended Queen's College, Oxford, where he received a bachelor's degree in physiology in 1954 and a medical degree in 1958. He completed an internship at Middlesex Hospital in London in 1959 and served as house surgeon of Queen Elizabeth Hospital in Birmingham in 1960. Sacks left England for the United States to accept an internship at Mount Zion Hospital in San Francisco (1961–62) before serving as a resident in neurology (1962–65) at the University of California, Los Angeles.

In 1965 Sacks became an instructor at Albert Einstein College of Medicine in the Bronx borough of New York City, eventually becoming a clinical professor of neurology (1966–75). He also joined Beth Abraham Hospital, a charity institution in the Bronx, as a staff neurologist (1966–2007). There he met a group of patients who had contracted a sleeping sickness, encephalitis lethargica, during an epidemic that broke out between 1917 and 1927. The patients had survived only to develop a type of parkinsonism that caused varying degrees of immobility, speechlessness, and depression. Sacks recounted the brief cure that the patients experienced after receiving the drug l-dopa and the drug's subsequent side effects in his 1973 book *Awakenings*, which was made into a motion picture in 1990.

Sacks enumerated further experiences, both professional and personal, in a series of volumes written for a popular audience. Having injured a leg in a mountaineering accident, he learned firsthand how a physician's dismissal of a patient's condition could hinder recuperation, a saga he related in *A Leg to Stand On* (1984). Sacks took care to illuminate the existential as well as pathological conditions of his patients in works such as *The Man Who Mistook His Wife for a Hat* (1986). While most critics found his descriptions of the often strange afflictions to be humane and sympathetic, some accused Sacks of merely attempting to excite and amuse his audience.

Sacks continued to record the extraordinary circumstances of the patients he encountered and the equally remarkable adaptations that they developed. In *Seeing Voices* (1989), he explored the ways in which sign language not only provides the deaf with a means of communication but also serves as the foundation for a discrete culture. In *An Anthropologist on Mars* (1995), he documented the lives of seven patients living with conditions ranging from autism to brain damage and described the unique ways in which they created functional lives in spite of their disabilities. Sacks described his journey to Micronesia to study a population with a high incidence of colour blindness and to Guam to study a mysterious form of paralysis in *The Island of the Colorblind* (1997). He presented further case studies in *The Mind Traveler* (1998), a program produced for television, and wrote of patients with conditions relating to music in *Musicophilia: Tales of Music and the Brain* (2007). *The Mind's Eye* (2010) investigated the compensatory mechanisms employed by people with sensory disorders, including himself (in the wake of vision loss in one eye due to ocular cancer). *Hallucinations* (2012) inventoried conditions and circumstances—from epilepsy to drug use to sensory deprivation—that can cause hallucinations and chronicled the effects of illusory neurological phenomena on those who experienced them. Among his autobiographical works were *Uncle Tungsten: Memories of a Chemical Boyhood* (2001), *Oaxaca Journal* (2002), and *On the Move* (2015). In 1989 Sacks received a Guggenheim fellowship for his studies of the influence of culture on the aberrant neurological processes underlying the rare inherited disease known as Tourette syndrome. In addition to his position at Beth Abraham, he served as

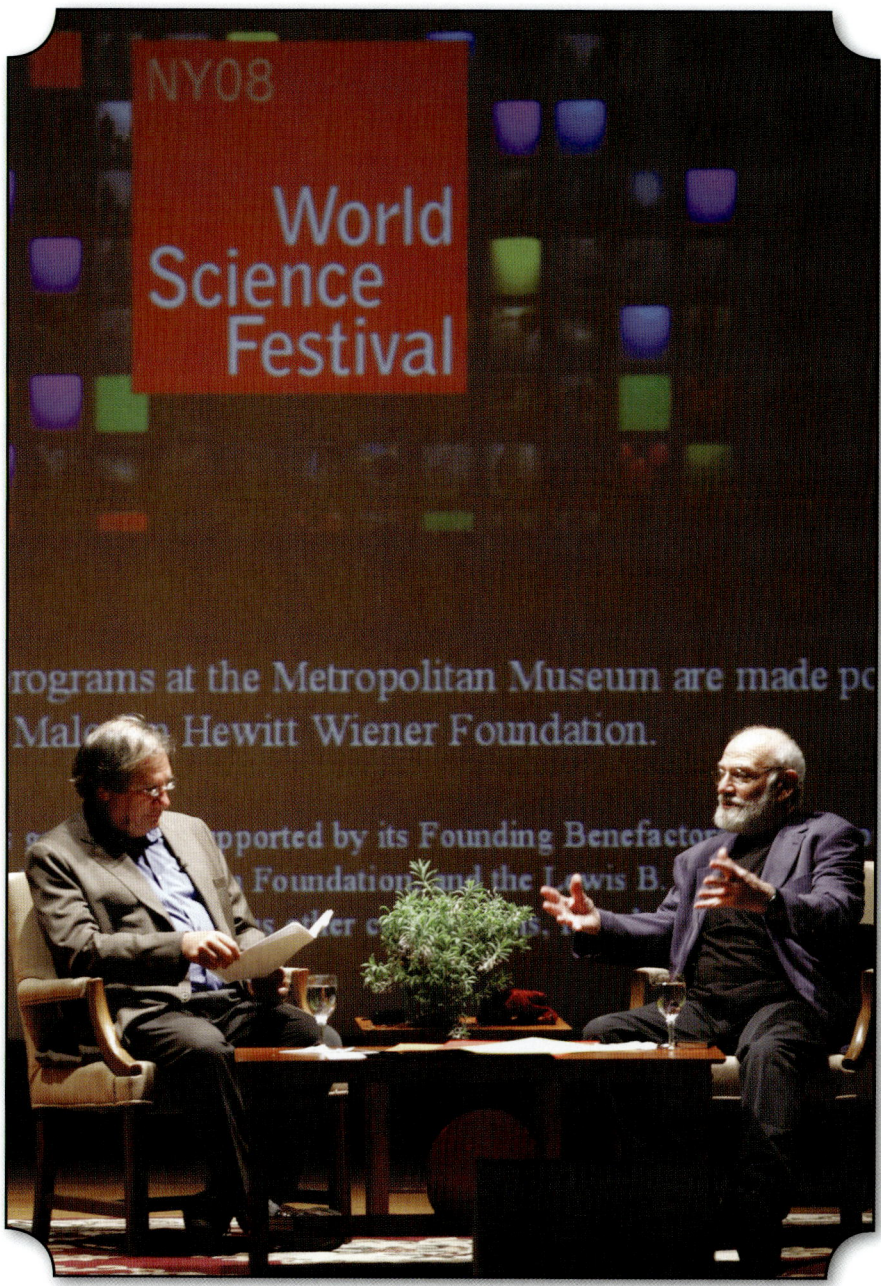

Oliver Sacks (right) *speaks at the 2008 World Science Festival in New York City.*

professor of neurology at the New York University School of Medicine (1992–2007) and the New York University Comprehensive Epilepsy Center (1999–2007). In 2007 Sacks became a professor of neurology and psychiatry at the Columbia University Medical Center in New York. He was also appointed Columbia University Artist, a position created for him to ensure that Columbia students from all disciplines would benefit from his association with the university. Sacks was made Commander of the British Empire (CBE) in 2008. Though he resided permanently in the United States, he never relinquished British citizenship. In February 2015 he announced that he had been diagnosed with terminal liver cancer. The ocular melanoma for which he had previously been treated spread to his liver, and he ultimately succumbed to the illness.

J. MICHAEL BISHOP
(born Feb. 22, 1936, York, Pa., U.S.)

J. Michael Bishop (in full John Michael Bishop) is an American virologist and co-winner (with Harold Varmus) of the Nobel Prize for Physiology or Medicine in 1989 for achievements in clarifying the origins of cancer.

Bishop graduated from Gettysburg College (Pennsylvania) in 1957 and from Harvard Medical School in 1962. After spending two years in internship and residency at Massachusetts General Hospital, Boston, he became a researcher in virology at the National Institutes of Health, Bethesda, Md. In 1968 he joined the faculty of the University of California Medical Center in San Francisco, becoming a full professor in 1972. From 1981 he also served as director of the university's George F. Hooper Research Foundation. In 1998 Bishop was elected chancellor of the University of California, San Francisco.

In 1970 Bishop teamed up with Varmus, and they set out to test the theory that healthy body cells contain dormant viral oncogenes that, when triggered, cause cancer. Working with the Rous sarcoma virus, known to cause cancer in chickens, Bishop and Varmus found that a gene similar to the cancer-causing gene within the virus was also present in healthy cells.

In 1976 Bishop and Varmus, together with two colleagues—Dominique Stehelin and Peter Vogt—published their findings, concluding that the virus had taken up the gene responsible for the cancer from a normal cell. After the virus had infected the cell and begun its usual process of replication, it incorporated the gene into its own genetic material. Subsequent research showed that such genes can cause cancer in several ways. Even without viral involvement, these genes can be converted by certain chemical carcinogens into a form that allows uncontrolled cellular growth.

Because the mechanism described by Bishop and Varmus seemed common to all forms of cancer, their work proved invaluable to cancer research. Today, scientists suspect that nearly 1 percent of the human genome, which contains an estimated 20,000 to 25,000 genes, is made up of proto-oncogenes—genes that when altered or mutated from their original form have the ability to cause cancer in animals.

Bishop was awarded the National Medal of Science in 2003. That same year, he published *How to Win the Nobel Prize: An Unexpected Life in Science*, a reflection on his life and work that also touches on historical aspects of science and on the intellectual environment of modern-day research.

HARALD ZUR HAUSEN
(born March 11, 1936, Gelsenkirchen, Germany)

Harald zur Hausen is a German virologist who was a corecipient, with Francoise Barré-Sinoussi and Luc Montagnier, of the 2008 Nobel Prize for Physiology or Medicine. Zur Hausen was given half the award in recognition of his discovery of the human papilloma virus (HPV) and its link to cervical cancer.

Zur Hausen received an M.D. in 1960 from the University of Düsseldorf, where he was a research fellow from 1962 to 1965; he continued in that capacity at the Children's Hospital of Philadelphia (1966–69). In the following years he worked in the virology departments of several German universities. In 1983 he was made scientific director and chairman of the German Cancer Research Center in Heidelberg; zur Hausen became emeritus professor there in 2003.

The discovery leading to zur Hausen's Nobel honour was made in the early 1980s. Though his findings were ill-supported at the time, they were later fully vindicated. His work led to the creation of the HPV vaccine, which significantly cuts the risk of developing cervical cancer, the second most common cancer among women.

HAROLD VARMUS
(born Dec. 18, 1939, Oceanside, N.Y., U.S.)

Harold Varmus (in full Harold Elliot Varmus) is an American virologist and cowinner (with J. Michael Bishop) of the Nobel Prize for Physiology or Medicine in 1989 for their work on the origins of cancer.

Varmus graduated from Amherst (Mass.) College (B.A.) in 1961, from Harvard University (M.A.) in 1962, and from Columbia University, New York City (M.D.), in

1966. He then joined the National Cancer Institute, Bethesda, Md., where he studied bacteria. In 1970 he went to the University of California, San Francisco, as a post-doctoral fellow. There he and Bishop began the research that was to win them the Nobel Prize.

Varmus and Bishop found that, under certain circumstances, normal genes in healthy cells of the body can cause cancer; these genes are called oncogenes. Oncogenes ordinarily control cellular growth and division, but, if they are picked up by infecting viruses or affected by chemical carcinogens, they can be rendered capable of causing cancer. This research, carried out with the aid of colleagues Dominique Stehelin and Peter Vogt in the mid-1970s, superseded a theory that cancer is caused by viral genes, distinct from a cell's normal genetic material, that lie dormant in body cells until activated by carcinogens.

Varmus remained on the faculty of the University of California, where he became a professor of biochemistry and biophysics in 1982. That same year he received an Albert Lasker Basic Medical Research Award for his investigations into the molecular genetics of cancer. He was director of the National Institutes of Health from 1993 to 1999, during which time he significantly increased the budget provided for research. In January 2000 Varmus was appointed president of Memorial Sloan-Kettering Cancer Center in New York City, and he subsequently founded the Public Library of Science (PLoS), a nonprofit organization dedicated to making medical and scientific literature freely available to the public. Varmus was a leading supporter of open-access journals and an advisor for Scientists and Engineers for America, a community of researchers and medical doctors committed to calling attention to science issues on a political level. In 2001 Varmus was awarded the National Medal of Science for his work on oncogenes and for his work to revitalize scientific research in the United States.

Varmus published numerous research papers throughout his career, was a coauthor of *Genes and the Biology of Cancer* (1993; with Robert A. Weinberg), and a coeditor of *Retroviruses* (1997; with John M. Coffin and Stephen H. Hughes).

FRANCOISE BARRÉ-SINOUSSI
(born July 30, 1947, Paris, France)

Francoise Barré-Sinoussi is a French virologist who was a corecipient, with Luc Montagnier and Harald zur Hausen, of the 2008 Nobel Prize for Physiology or Medicine. She and Montagnier shared half the prize for their work in identifying the human immunodeficiency virus (HIV), the cause of acquired immunodeficiency syndrome (AIDS).

Barré-Sinoussi earned a Ph.D. (1975) at the Pasteur Institute in Garches, France, and did postdoctoral work in the United States at the National Cancer Institute in Bethesda, Md. In 1975 she joined the Pasteur Institute in Paris, and in 1996 she became head of the Retrovirus Biology Unit (later called Regulation of Retroviral Infections Unit) there.

When Montagnier led

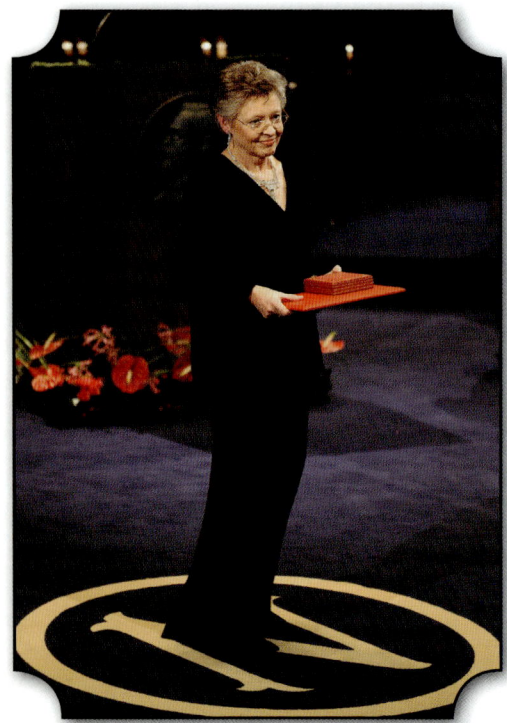

Francoise Barré-Sinoussi receives the 2008 Nobel Prize for Physiology or Medicine in Stockholm, Sweden.

efforts at the Pasteur Institute in 1982 to determine a cause for AIDS, Barré-Sinoussi was a member of his team. Through dissection of an infected patient's lymph node, they determined that AIDS was caused by a retrovirus, which came to be known as HIV. Their work led to the development of new antiviral drugs and diagnostic methods.

FRANCIS COLLINS
(born April 14, 1950, Staunton, Va., U.S.)

Francis Collins (in full Francis Sellers Collins) is an American geneticist who discovered genes causing genetic diseases and led the U.S. National Institutes of Health (NIH) public research consortium in the Human

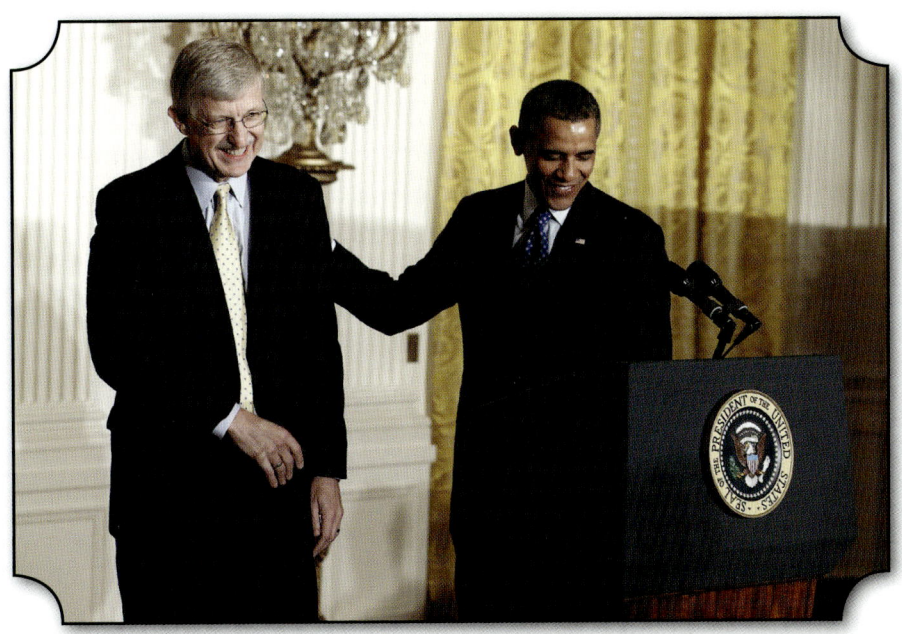

Francis Collins stands with U.S. Pres. Barack Obama as he announces the BRAIN Initiative, a collaboration between the NIH and other organizations.

Genome Project (HGP). In 2009 Pres. Barack Obama nominated Collins to head the NIH, a move that was confirmed by the U.S. Senate in August of that year.

Homeschooled by his mother for much of his childhood, Collins took an early interest in science. He received a B.S. from the University of Virginia (1970), went on to Yale University to earn an M.S. and a Ph.D. (1974), and earned an M.D. (1977) at the University of North Carolina at Chapel Hill. In 1984 Collins joined the staff of the University of Michigan at Ann Arbor as an assistant professor. His work at Michigan would earn him a reputation as one of the world's foremost genetics researchers. In 1989 he announced the discovery of the gene that causes cystic fibrosis. The following year a Collins-led team found the gene that causes neurofibromatosis, a genetic disorder that generates the growth of tumours. He also served as a leading researcher in a collaboration of six laboratories that in 1993 uncovered the gene that causes Huntington chorea, a neurological disease.

Prior to the HGP, the base sequences of numerous human genes had been determined through contributions made by many individual scientists. However, the vast majority of the human genome remained unexplored, and researchers, having recognized the necessity and value of having at hand the basic information of the human genomic sequence, were beginning to search for ways to uncover this information more quickly. Because the HGP required billions of dollars that would inevitably be taken away from traditional biomedical research, many scientists, politicians, and ethicists became involved in vigorous debates over the merits, risks, and relative costs of sequencing the entire human genome in one concerted undertaking. Despite the controversy, the Human Genome Project was initiated in 1990 under Collins's leadership, with support from the U.S. Department of

Energy and the National Institutes of Health (NIH). The effort was soon joined by scientists from around the world. Moreover, a series of technical advances in the sequencing process itself and in the computer hardware and software used to track and analyze the resulting data enabled rapid progress of the project.

In 1993 Collins, by then a full professor, left Michigan to take the post as head of the National Human Genome Research Institute (NHGRI) of the NIH, which had begun work on the HGP three years earlier with a stated goal of completing the sequencing project in 15 years at a cost of $3 billion by coordinating the work of a number of leading academic research centres around the country, in collaboration with the U.S. Department of Energy and the Wellcome Trust of London. Driven by a sincere interest in successful research that could help humanity, Collins was an obvious choice for the job, and he willingly took a sizable pay cut to participate in a historic project.

The necessity of a government effort was questioned when a rival operation, Celera Genomics, emerged in 1998 and appeared to be working even faster than the HGP at deciphering the DNA sequence. Headed by American geneticist and businessman J. Craig Venter, a former NIH scientist, Celera had devised its own, quicker method—though some scientists, Collins among them, questioned the accuracy of the work. However, in the end the public and private endeavours came together. On June 26, 2000, Collins, Venter, and U.S. Pres. Bill Clinton gathered in Washington, D.C., to announce that the rough draft sequence of the DNA in the human genetic map had been completed through the combined effort of Collins's public research consortium and Venter's private company. The breakthrough was hailed as the first step toward helping doctors diagnose, treat, and even prevent thousands of illnesses caused by genetic disorders. In April 2003, following further analysis of the sequence, the HGP came to a close. The announcement of the completion of the HGP coincided with the 50th anniversary of American geneticist and biophysicist James D. Watson and British biophysicist Francis Crick's publication on the structure of DNA.

A practicing Christian, Collins freely expressed the awe he experienced as a leader in the uncloaking of one of the mysteries of life. As concerns arose about the moral and ethical implications of the research he had conducted, Collins actively cautioned against misuse of genetic information. At congressional hearings in July 2000, Collins urged the passage of federal law to set guidelines on how individuals' genetic information could be handled. "The potential for mischief is quite great," he said. On Aug. 1, 2008, Collins resigned from his position as director of the NHGRI in order to pursue broader, more flexible research opportunities. In October 2009, following his Senate confirmation to head the NIH, Collins was appointed by Pope Benedict XVI to the Pontifical Academy of Sciences, an organization that promotes advancement in the fundamental understanding of scientific questions and the investigation of ethical and philosophical issues associated with science.

JAMES THOMSON

(born Dec. 20, 1958, Chicago, Ill., U.S.)

James Thomson (in full James Alexander Thomson) is an American biologist who was among the first to isolate human embryonic stem cells and the first to transform human skin cells into stem cells.

Thomson grew up in the Chicago suburb of Oak Park. At the University of Illinois, from which he graduated in 1981 with a bachelor's degree in biophysics, Thomson was encouraged to work in the biology laboratories, where he became interested in the process of early development—the explosive surge of biological activity that occurs when a fertilized egg implants itself in a womb and then begins to divide and form the specialized cells that eventually become the great variety of tissues in the body. He continued his education and research at the University of Pennsylvania, where he gained a doctorate in veterinary medicine in 1985 and a doctorate in molecular biology in 1988. Thomson then completed a postdoctoral fellowship at the Oregon Regional Primate Center (1989–91).

In 1991 Thomson moved to the University of Wisconsin, where he continued his research at the Wisconsin Regional Primate Centre. Having learned in 1980 that biologists had succeeded in extracting embryonic stem cells from mice, Thomson decided to conduct stem cell research on a species much more similar to humans, the rhesus monkey. Embryonic stem cells are derived from the inner cell mass of a mammalian embryo at a very early stage of development, when it is composed of a hollow sphere of dividing cells (a blastocyst). After many months of painstaking work, he succeeded in isolating the rhesus monkey embryonic stem cells in 1995. That same year he was appointed chief pathologist of the primate centre. The obvious next step, to Thomson, was to try to extract stem cells from human embryos. However, this confronted him with a moral dilemma, as such an extraction is fatal to the embryo. After consulting with several bioethicists at the university, Thomson decided that continued research was ethical as long as the embryos, created by couples who no longer wanted them in order to have children, would otherwise be destroyed. In 1998 he successfully isolated stem cells from a human embryo, almost simultaneously with researchers at Johns Hopkins University. Thomson was appointed scientific director of the WiCell Research Institute, affiliated with the

University of Wisconsin, in 1999.

Thomson had assigned the patent for his discovery, which covered both the method of isolating the cells and the cells themselves, to the Wisconsin Alumni Research Foundation. When U.S. Pres. George W. Bush announced in August 2001 that the federal government would only support research on the 64 existing lines (self-sustaining colonies) of human embryonic stem cells, the National Institutes of Health, the agency responsible for implementing the decision, was forced to negotiate with the foundation in order to gain access to the stem cells. Thomson, though disappointed that the Bush edict restricted the creation of new cell lines, was generally pleased that his research could go forward. By November 2007 his team had transformed human skin cells into stem cells—called induced pluripotent stem cells (iPS)—through the insertion of four genes.

Thomson also became an adjunct professor at the University of California, Santa Barbara, in 2007. He was appointed director of regenerative biology at the Morgridge Institute for Research in Madison, Wis., in 2008.

SHINYA YAMANAKA
(born Sept. 4, 1962, Osaka, Japan)

Shinya Yamanaka (Japanese Yamanaka Shinya) is a Japanese physician and researcher who developed a revolutionary method for generating stem cells from existing cells of the body. This method involved inserting specific genes into the nuclei of adult cells (e.g., connective-tissue cells), a process that resulted in the reversion of cells from an adult state to a pluripotent state. As pluripotent cells, they had regained the capacity to differentiate into any cell type of the body. Thus, the reverted cells became known as induced

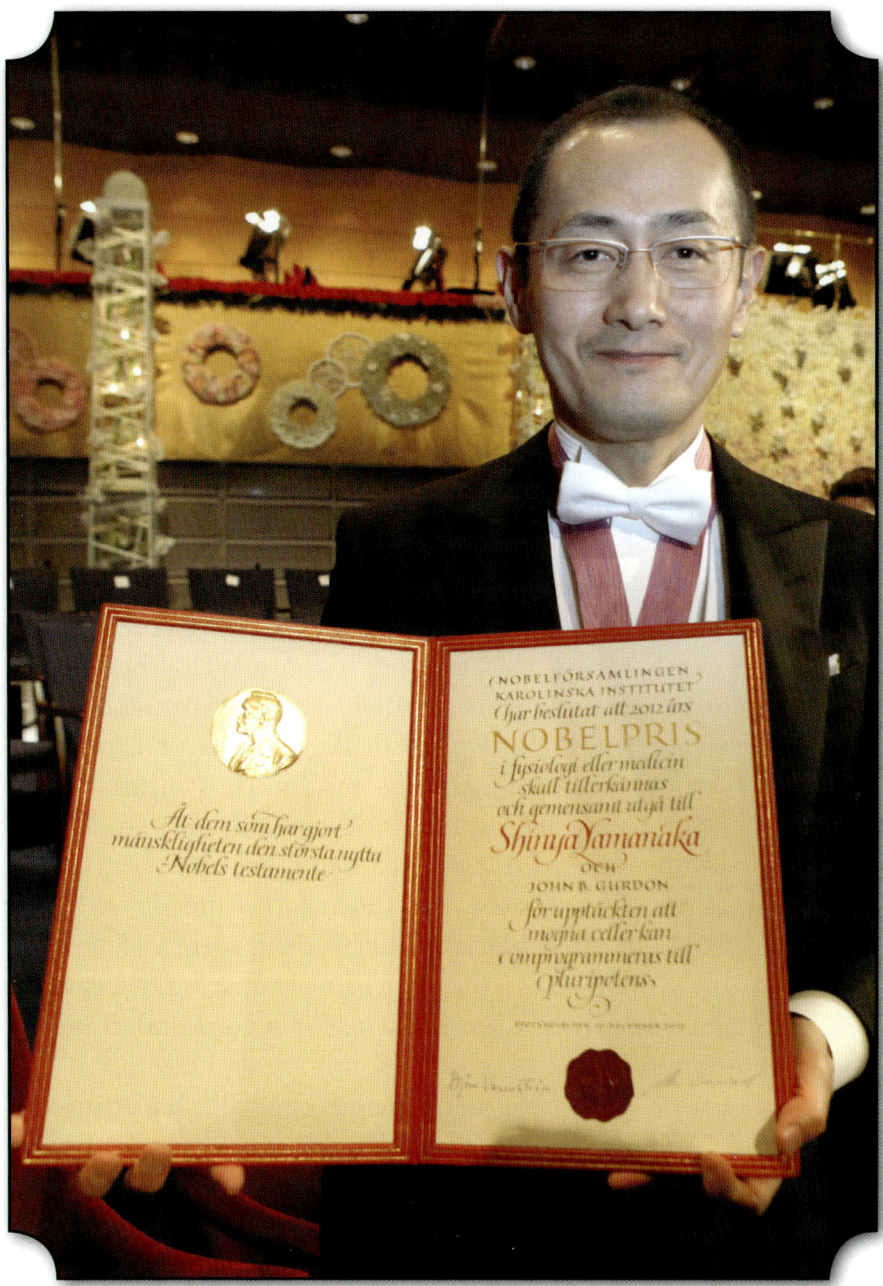

Shinya Yamanaka stands with his 2012 Nobel Prize in Physiology or Medicine, which he shared with John B. Gurdon, in Stockholm, Sweden.

pluripotent stem (iPS) cells. Yamanaka and British developmental biologist John B. Gurdon shared the 2012 Nobel Prize for Physiology or Medicine for the discovery that mature cells could be reprogrammed.

Yamanaka received an M.D. from Kobe University in 1987 and a Ph.D. in pharmacology from the Osaka City University Graduate School in 1993. That year he joined the Gladstone Institute of Cardiovascular Disease, San Francisco, where he began investigating the *c-Myc* gene in different strains of knockout mice (mice in which a specific gene has been rendered nonfunctional in order to investigate the gene's function). In 1996 Yamanaka returned to Osaka City University, where he remained until 1999, when he took a position at the Nara Institute of Science and Technology. During this period his research became increasingly focused on stem cells. In 2004 he moved to the Institute for Frontier Medical Sciences at Kyoto University, where he began his landmark studies on finding ways to induce pluripotency in cells. Yamanaka again sought research opportunities in the United States and subsequently was awarded funding that allowed him to split his time between Kyoto and the Gladstone Institute of Cardiovascular Disease. Yamanaka became a senior investigator at the Gladstone Institute in 2007.

In 2006 Yamanaka announced that he had succeeded in generating iPS cells. The cells had the properties of embryonic stem cells but were produced by inserting four specific genes into the nuclei of mouse adult fibroblasts (connective-tissue cells). The following year Yamanaka reported that he had derived iPS cells from human adult fibroblasts—the first successful attempt at generating human versions of these cells.

This discovery marked a turning point in stem-cell research, because it offered a way of obtaining human stem cells without the controversial use of human embryos. Yamanaka's technique to convert adult cells into iPS cells up to that time had employed a retrovirus that contained the *c-Myc* gene. This gene was believed to play a fundamental role in reprogramming the nuclei of adult cells. However, Yamanaka recognized that the activation of *c-Myc* during the process of creating iPS cells led to the formation of tumours when the stem cells were later transplanted into mice. He subsequently created iPS cells without *c-Myc* in order to render the cells noncancerous and thereby overcome a major concern in the therapeutic safety of iPS cells. In 2008 Yamanaka reported another breakthrough—the generation of iPS cells from mouse liver and stomach cells.

Yamanaka received multiple awards for his contributions to stem-cell research, including the Robert Koch Prize (2008), the Shaw Prize in Life Science and Medicine (2008), the Gairdner Foundation International Award (2009), the Albert Lasker Basic Medical Research Award (2009), and the Millennium Technology Prize (2012).

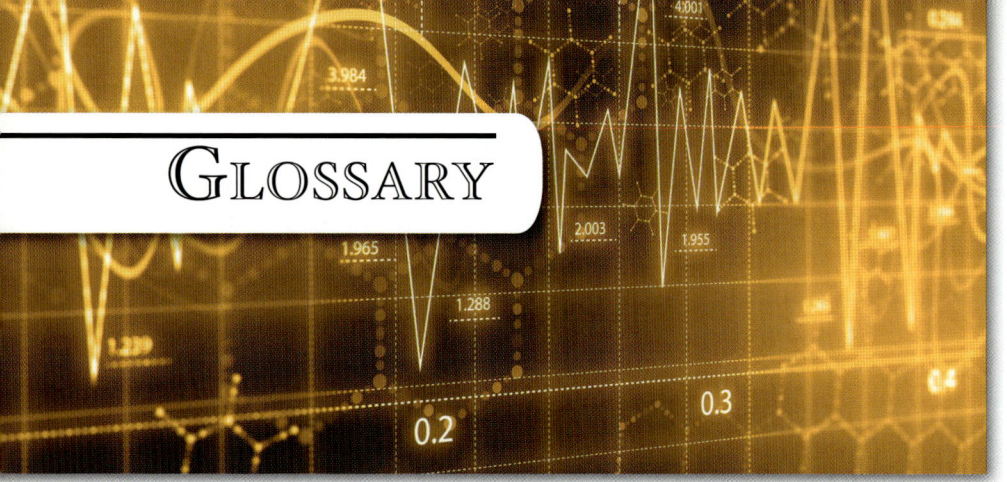

Glossary

acupuncture A method of relieving pain or curing illness by placing needles into a person's skin at particular points on the body.

agglutination A reaction in which particles (e.g., red blood cells or bacteria) suspended in a liquid collect into clumps and which occurs especially as a serologic response to a specific antibody.

anastomosis The surgical union of parts and especially hollow tubular parts.

antibody A substance produced by the body to fight disease.

auscultation The act of listening to sounds arising within organs (e.g., the lungs) as an aid to diagnosis and treatment.

binaural Of, relating to, or involving two or both ears.

bloodletting Bleeding induced for transfusion, apheresis, diagnostic testing, or experimental procedures and widely used in the past to treat many types of disease but now limited to the treatment of only a few specific conditions.

cathode ray The high-speed electrons emitted in a stream from the heated cathode of a vacuum tube.

chordate Any of a phylum (Chordata) of animals having at least at some stage of development of a notochord, dorsally situated central nervous system, and gill clefts and including the vertebrates, lancelets, and tunicates.

ciliate A single-celled organism that, at some stage in its life cycle, possesses cilia, short hairlike organelles used for locomotion and food gathering.

defibrillator A device that gives an electric shock to a person's heart in order to make it beat normally again, especially after a heart attack.

DNA Short for deoxyribonucleic acid. Any of various nucleic acids that are usually the molecular basis of heredity, are constructed of a double helix held together by hydrogen bonds between purine and pyrimidine bases which project inward from two chains containing alternate links of deoxyribose and phosphate, and that in eukaryotes are localized chiefly in cell nuclei.

empiricism The practice of relying on observation and experiment, especially in the natural sciences.

epidemiology A branch of medical science that deals with the incidence, distribution, and control of disease in a population.

flagellate Any of a group of protozoans, mostly uninucleate organisms, that possess, at some time in the life cycle, one to many flagella for locomotion and sensation. (A flagellum is a hairlike structure capable of whiplike lashing movements that furnish locomotion.)

germ theory In medicine, the theory that certain diseases are caused by the invasion of the body by microorganisms.

growth factor A substance (e.g., vitamin B12 or an interleukin) that promotes growth and especially cellular growth.

humour One of the four fluids entering into the constitution of the body and determining by their relative proportions a person's health and temperament. In the ancient physiological theory still current in the European Middle Ages and later, the four cardinal humours were blood, phlegm, choler (yellow bile), and melancholy (black bile).

hydrotherapy The therapeutic use of water (e.g., in a whirlpool bath).

passive immunity Immunity acquired by transfer of antibodies (e.g., by injection of serum from an individual with active immunity).

pessary A device worn in the vagina to support the uterus, remedy a malposition, or prevent conception.

pluripotent Capable of differentiating into one of many cell types.

pneuma Soul or spirit.

polarization The action or process of affecting radiation and especially light so that the vibrations of the wave assume a definite form.

puerperal Of, relating to, or occurring during childbirth or the period immediately following.

purgative A medicine or food that causes the bowels to empty.

radioimmunoassay A test used to detect the presence or quantity of a substance (e.g., a protein) based on its capacity to act as an antigen of a substance that has been radioactively labeled.

resect To surgically remove part or all of an organ or structure.

side chain A branched chain of atoms attached to the principal chain or to a ring in a molecule.

stem cell A type of cell in the body that is able to develop into any one of various kinds of cells (e.g., blood cells and skin cells).

transection A transverse cut.

transposon A transposable element, especially when it contains genetic material controlling functions other

than those related to its relocation.
virulence The relative capacity of a pathogen to overcome body defenses.
viscera Internal organs of the body, especially one (e.g., the heart, liver, or intestine) located in the great cavity of the trunk proper.
vivisection The cutting of or operation on a living animal usually for physiological or pathological investigation.

For Further Reading

Aldridge, Susan. *Trailblazers in Medicine*. New York, NY: Rosen Publishing, 2015.

Belofsky, Nathan. *Strange Medicine: A Shocking History of Real Medical Practices Through the Ages*. New York, NY: Penguin, 2013.

Butterfield, Moira, and Pat Jacobs. *The Human Body*. New York, NY: Cavendish Square, 2016.

Farndon, John, and Alex Woolf, Anne Rooney, and Liz Gogerly. *Great Scientists*. New York, NY: Rosen Publishing, 2013.

Harris, Michael C. *Unusual Diseases*. Tarrytown, NY: Marshall Cavendish, 2011.

Hollar, Sherman, ed. *Pioneers in Medicine: From the Classical World to Today*. New York: Britannica Educational Publishing, 2013.

Johnson, Rose. *Discoveries in Medicine that Changed the World*. New York, NY: Rosen Publishing, 2015.

Le Fanu, James. *The Rise and Fall of Modern Medicine*. New York, NY: Basic Books, 2012.

Luchetti, Cathy. *Medicine Women: The Story of Early-American Women Doctors*. New York, NY: Crown, 1998.

Marshall Cavendish Reference. *Diseases, Disorders, and Injuries*. Tarrytown, NY: Marshall Cavendish, 2011.

Marshall Cavendish Reference. *Human Body from A to Z*. Tarrytown, NY: Marshall Cavendish, 2012.

Morrison, Heather S. *Inventors of Health and Medical*

Technology. New York, NY: Cavendish Square, 2015.

Nutton, Vivian. *Ancient Medicine*. New York, NY: Routledge, 2013.

Oxlade, Chris. *Top Ten Scientific Discoveries that Changed the World*. New York, NY: Rosen Publishing, 2010.

Parker, Steve. *Kill or Cure: An Illustrated History of Medicine*. New York, NY: DK Publishing, 2013.

Pickover, Clifford A. *The Medical Book: From Witch Doctors to Robot Surgeons, 250 Milestones in the History of Medicine*. New York, NY: Sterling, 2012.

Porter, Roy. *The Greatest Benefit to Mankind: A Medical History of Humanity*. New York, NY: W.W. Norton, 1998.

Rogers, Kara, ed. *Battling and Managing Disease*. New York, NY: Britannica Educational Publishing, 2011.

Rogers, Kara, ed. *Infectious Diseases*. New York, NY: Britannica Educational Publishing, 2011.

Rogers, Kara, ed. *Medicine and Healers Through History*. New York, NY: Britannica Educational Publishing, 2011.

Rooney, Anne. *The History of Medicine*. New York, NY: Rosen Publishing, 2013.

Wanjie, Anne. *The Basics of the Human Body*. New York, NY: Rosen Publishing, 2014.

Wolfe, James, ed. *Genetic Testing and Gene Therapy*. New York, NY: Britannica Educational Publishing, 2016.

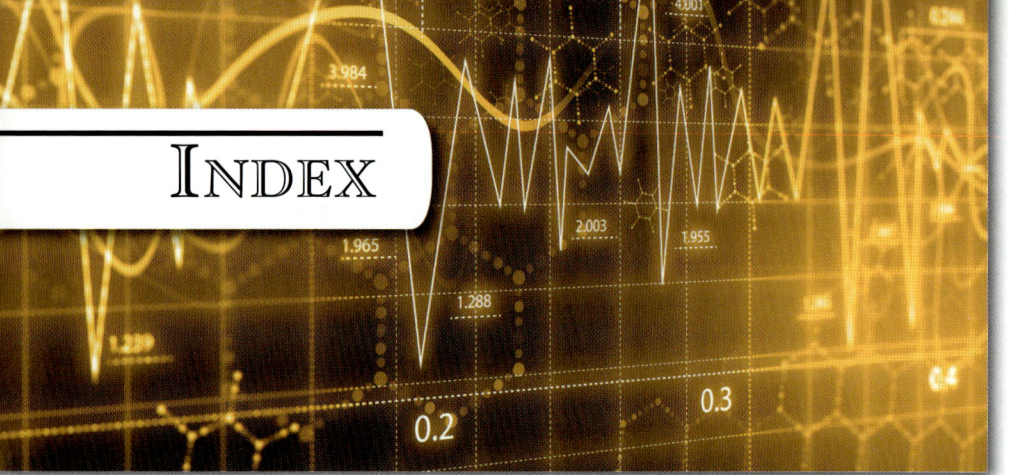

Index

A

American Red Cross, 138, 140–141
amputation, as fracture treatment, 89
analytic psychology, 225–230
anaphylaxis, 108
anatomy, first textbook, 62, 64–65
anthrax
  discovery of disease cycle, 164–166
  vaccination, 149–150
antisepsis, 115, 117, 118, 154, 155–157
Apgar, Virginia, 259–262
Apgar Score System, 259, 261–262
Avery, Oswald, 230–232, 283
Avicenna, 41–50, 57, 59

B

bacteriology, founding of science of, 164–170
Baker, Sara Josephine, 223–225
Banting, Frederick Grant, 242–244, 247, 248
Barnard, Christiaan, 267, 273–275
Barré-Sinoussi, Francoise, 285, 286, 292, 294–295
Barton, Clara, 138–141
Bateson, William, 216–218
Bearn, Alexander Gordon, 276–279
Behring, Emil von, 186, 189–190
Best, Charles, 242, 243, 247–248
birth control, 232, 234–236
Bishop, J. Michael, 290–291, 292, 293
Blackwell, Elizabeth, 129–131, 162
Blalock, Alfred, 245, 248–249
Blalock-Taussig shunt, 246
blindness, early surgical treatment for, 88
bloodletting, 97, 98
blood transfusions, preservation of blood for, 253
blood typing, development of, 219, 220
"blue baby" syndrome, 244, 245–246, 248–249
Blumberg, Baruch S., 280–281
Book of the Cure, 41, 43, 44
Book on Medical Discourses, A, 159, 160
Broad Street pump outbreak,

109, 110–111
bubonic plague, discovery of causative organism, 182–183

C

cancer
  and occupational exposure, 88, 90
  origins of, 290, 291, 292, 293
Canon of Medicine, The, 41, 45–47, 49
Chain, Ernst Boris, 237, 240, 246, 247, 255
Cheselden, William, 87–88, 93
chloroform, 110, 115
cholera, 109, 110–112, 149, 164, 168–169
circulation, first recognition of full body, 67, 70–74
Civilization and Its Discontents, 211
Cleveland, Emeline Horton, 158–159
Cohen, Stanley, 259, 275–276
collective unconscious, 226, 228
Collins, Francis, 295–298
Cooley, Denton A., 271
Crick, Francis Harry Compton, 265–267, 270, 282, 283, 298
Crimean War, 123, 125–127
Crumpler, Rebecca Lee, 159–160

D

defibrillators, 262, 263
De Materia Medica, 32
deoxyribonucleic acid (DNA)
  discovery as basis of heredity, 230, 232, 283
  discovery of molecular structure of, 265–266, 269, 270, 282, 283, 298
diphtheria, prevention of, 182, 186, 189, 216
disease, cell theory of, 131–132, 134–136
Diseases, 27
Division of Child Hygiene, 223–225
Dorsey, Rebecca Lee, 215–216
double helix, 270, 283
Drew, Charles Richard, 253–255

E

Ehrlich, Paul, 183–188, 189, 238
Embassy, The, 28
encephalitis lethargica, 287
endocrinology, 215
endorphins, 280
Epidemics, 27
epidemiology, founding of study, 109, 110–112, 178–180
epidermal growth factor, 276
ether, first public demonstration of, 122

F

Fabrica, 64–65
Fallopius, Gabriel, 66–67
fermentation, 141, 144–145
Fleming, Alexander, 236–241, 246, 247, 255
Flexner, Abraham, 218–219
Florey, Howard Walter, 237, 240, 246–247, 255
foxglove, 94, 95–96, 97
Franklin, Rosalind, 266, 269–270
Freud, Sigmund, 190–213, 226, 227, 228

G

Galen, 30, 31, 32–38, 47, 49, 57, 59, 63, 65, 66, 67
genetics, founding of field, 216–218
Geneva Convention, 138, 140
germ theory of disease, early proponents of, 111, 149, 157
gonorrhea, 93–94
Great Surgery Book, 56, 59–60
Guillemin, Roger Charles Louis, 271, 279–280, 281, 282

H

Harvey, William, 37, 67–76, 80, 82
heart
  first artificial heart implant, 271
  first human heart transplant in the United States, 267
  first human heart transplant in the world, 267, 273, 274
  first surgery, 214
hepatitis B, 280, 281
hernias, 62
Hippocrates, 25–31, 35, 36, 40, 47
Hippocratic Oath, 25, 28–30
histology, founding of field, 78, 79–80, 81
Hua Tuo, 38–40
Human Genome Project, 295–298
human immunodeficiency virus (HIV), 285, 286, 294, 295
human papilloma virus (HPV), 292
Hunter, John, 93–94
hypothalamus gland, 279, 282

I

Imhotep, 23–25
insulin, 242, 243, 247, 248, 255, 272
Interpretation of Dreams, The, 197–199

J

Jacobi, Mary Putnam, 162–163
Jenner, Edward, 99–104, 150
Julian, Percy, 249–251
Jung, Carl, 61, 205, 210, 225–230

K

Kantrowitz, Adrian, 267
Koch, Robert, 149, 164–170, 172, 184

L

Laënnec, René-Théophile-Hyacinthe, 104–108
Landsteiner, Karl, 219–221
Laveran, Alphonse, 171–172
Leeuwenhoek, Antonie van, 82–87
Levi-Montalcini, Rita, 257–259, 275
Lind, James, 91–92
Lister, Joseph, 118, 153–158
lysozome, 239, 240, 247

M

mafeisan, 38
Magendie, François, 108
Maimonides, Moses, 51–55
malaria, 77, 171–172
Malpighi, Marcello, 78–82, 83, 85
Mayo, Charles Horace, 120, 121
Mayo, Charles William, 121

Mayo, William James, 119–120, 121
Mayo, William Worrall, 119
McClintock, Barbara, 251–253
Medical Inquiries and Observations upon the Diseases of the Mind, 99
miasmas, 111, 156, 169, 172
microscopes, early use of, 78, 79–80, 81, 83–87
Mishna, 51, 53, 54
mobile genetic elements, 251, 252–253
molecular asymmetry, 141, 142–143
Montagnier, Luc, 285–286, 292, 294
Morton, William Thomas Green, 122–123
Moses and Monotheism, 212–213
Murray, Joseph E., 268–269

N

neuron, discovery of, 180–181
nerve-growth factor, 259, 275
Nightingale, Florence, 123–129, 131
nitrous oxide, 114–115
nursing, formalizing of education for, 123, 128

O

Origin and Development of Psychoanalysis, 205
Osler, William, 25, 50, 173–176

P

pacemakers, 262, 263
Paracelsus, 56–61
Paré, Ambroise, 61–62
Pasteur, Louis, 141–153, 156, 165, 166, 172
pasteurization, 141, 145
Pedanius Dioscorides, 31–32
penicillin, 236, 237, 239–240, 241, 246, 247, 255
phantom limb syndrome, 62
Planned Parenthood, 234, 235
polio vaccine, 221, 256–257, 263, 264
Pott, Percivall, 88–91
Pott disease, 90–91
Preston, Ann, 112–114
Principles and Practice of Medicine, 173, 174–175
proprietas, 48
psychoanalysis, founding of, 190–213
Psychopathology of Everyday Life, The, 199–200
puerperal fever, 115–117, 118, 216
purging, 97, 98

Q

quinine, 172

R

rabies vaccination, 150–151
radioimmunoassay, 271–272
Ramón y Cajal, Santiago, 180–181
Rāzī, al-, 40–41, 49, 50
reduction, as fracture treatment, 89
Reed, Walter, 176–180
Rötgen, Wilhelm, Conrad, 170–171
Rush, Benjamin, 97–99

S

Sabin, Albert, 256–257
Sabin, Florence Rena, 221–223
Sacks, Oliver, 286–290
Salk, Jonas, 256, 263–265
Safford, Mary Jane, 160–161
Sanger, Margaret, 232–235, 236
Schally, Andrew V., 271, 279, 281–282
scurvy, 91–92
Semmelweis, Ignaz Philipp, 115–118
serum therapy, 182, 186, 189
Shibasaburo, Kitasato, 181–183, 189
side chain theory of immunity, 185–186
silkworm crisis, 146, 148
smallpox vaccination, 99, 100–104, 150
Snow, John, 109–112, 168
soybeans, 249
spinal nerves, 108
spontaneous generation, 82, 85–86, 145–146
stem cells
  embryonic, 298, 299–300
  induced pluripotent, 300, 302–303
stethoscope, invention of, 104, 106–107
Stopes, Marie, 235–236
streptomycin, 241, 242
Sydenham, Thomas, 76–78
Sydenham chorea, 76–77
syphilis, 56, 60, 62, 93, 183, 187–188, 221, 238

T

Taussig, Helen Brooke, 244–246
tetanus, prevention of, 181, 182, 189
Thomson, James, 298–300
Three Essays on the Theory of Sexuality, 200, 208
Totem and Taboo, 209, 210
transplant rejection, 268
tuberculosis
  discovery of bacteria, 164, 167–168, 169, 184
  treatment for, 241, 242

V

variolation, 101
Varmus, Harold, 290, 292–294
Vesalius, Andreas, 37, 62–66, 67
Virchow, Rudolf, 131–137
virulence, Pasteur's theory of, 152, 153
vivisection, 34–35

W

Waksman, Selman Abraham, 241–242
Watson, James Dewey, 265, 266, 270, 282–285, 298
Wells, Horace, 114–115
Wilkins, Maurice, 265, 266, 282
Williams, Daniel Hale, 214–215
Wilson disease, 276, 277–278
Withering, William, 94–97
women
  first female doctor, 129–131
  first major surgery performed by a woman, 159

X

X-rays, discovery of, 170–171

Y

Yalow, Rosalyn S., 271–273, 279, 281
Yamanaka, Shinya, 300–303
yellow fever, 176, 178–180

Z

Zoll, Paul Maurice, 262–263
zur Hausen, Harald, 285, 292, 294